Hysterosalpingography
and Pelvic Ultrasound
Imaging in Infertility and Gynecology

Hysterosalpingography and Pelvic Ultrasound
Imaging in Infertility and Gynecology

Isabel C. Yoder, M.D.
Assistant Professor of
Radiology, Harvard Medical
School; Radiologist,
Department of Radiology,
Uroradiology Section,
Massachusetts General
Hospital, Boston,
Massachusetts

Foreword by
Alvin M. Siegler, M.D.,
D.Sc.
Clinical Professor,
Department of Obstetrics and
Gynecology,
State University of New York
Health Sciences Center at
Brooklyn, Brooklyn,
New York

Illustrations by
Edith Tagrin
Chief, Medical Art Unit,
Massachusetts General
Hospital, Boston,
Massachusetts

Little, Brown
and Company
Boston/Toronto

Library of Congress Catalog Card No. 88-81927

ISBN 0-316-96881-1

Printed in the United States of America

MV

To my parents, Lino and Hélène Saldaña

Contents

Foreword

It has been a privilege and an honor to have been asked to write the foreword to this excellent book, which should serve both gynecologists and radiologists as a source for the latest information on hysterosalpingography.

Hysterosalpingography and Pelvic Ultrasound: Imaging in Infertility and Gynecology, by Isabel C. Yoder, M.D., is written in a clear and concise fashion. It is logically divided into three main subjects beginning with a description of the technique of hysterosalpingography, following with its use for the detection of tubal abnormalities, and concluding with a comprehensive review of its value in the management of congenital uterine anomalies and intrauterine defects.

Dr. Yoder uses the balloon catheter technique very effectively for most of the studies presented and correctly stresses the importance of fluoroscopic monitoring and spot film radiographs. The new technique of selective salpingography is described as an attempt to overcome instances of proximal tubal obstruction.

The chapters on the fallopian tube include discussions and appropriate radiographs showing the abnormalities associated with proximal and distal tubal obstruction and their differential diagnoses. The salpingograms showing the end results of the different types of tubal sterilization are especially interesting. Dr. Yoder properly stresses the need for the post-drainage film to detect peritubal adhesions.

The concluding chapter, an outstanding one, is devoted to abnormalities of the uterine cavity detected by hysterography. Every variety of congenital uterine anomaly that can be seen radiographically is illustrated. The value of hysterography in the management of abnormal uterine bleeding is revealed by the illustrations of various submucosal lesions.

The author has succeeded, without a doubt, in updating the subject of hysterosalpingography by including relevant references, almost all of which were written since 1980. Clear illustrations of the abnormalities detected by this radiologic procedure are accompanied by detailed legends, as needed, so that the clinical picture is complete, making this book much more than an atlas on hysterosalpingography. Dr. Yoder uses sonograms with corresponding labeled schematics to improve the evaluation of a finding. When necessary to complete a topic, Dr. Yoder has secured the best available illustrations.

After reading this fine book, one can conclude only that a carefully performed and properly interpreted hysterosalpingogram should remain an important diagnostic procedure to be used in conjunction with sonography and pelvic endoscopy in properly selected patients.

Alvin M. Siegler, M.D., D.Sc.

Preface

This book is intended to be a standard text on hysterosalpingography. It will serve radiologists and gynecologists as a complete guide to the performance and interpretation of the hysterosalpingogram. The book is based on fourteen years of clinical experience and over one thousand hysterosalpingograms performed and correlated with the results of laparoscopy, surgery, or biopsy.

Hysterosalpingography and Pelvic Ultrasound: Imaging in Infertility and Gynecology is divided into three major subjects. The first emphasizes techniques and normal variations, the second covers tubal pathology and surgery, and the third includes all uterine malformations and abnormalities leading to distortion of the uterine cavity. Throughout the book hysterosalpingography is correlated with transabdominal sonography so that in each topic diagnostically complementary views of the female genital tract are included. Thus, for the first time these two radiologic studies are integrated into a single text for the use of both gynecologists and radiologists. Moreover, all of the sonograms shown in the book have adjacent labeled drawings so that they can be readily interpreted.

The majority of patients undergoing hysterosalpingograms are women experiencing infertility. Current medical advances in this field and social factors affecting it ensure that the demand for hysterosalpingography will continue to increase. For example, the application of microsurgical techniques to fallopian tube surgery doubles the success rate of the operation. Pre- and postoperative evaluation of the tubes can best be achieved with the hysterosalpingogram, the only procedure available that delineates the inner lumen of the tubes. The present trend to postpone childbearing while women establish careers and the rising rate of venereal infections increase women's risk of tubal obstruction and subsequent infertility. In addition, because of the increasing difficulty in adopting babies women will more likely choose to undergo complex surgery to reverse tubal obstruction, especially since new techniques offer a better chance of eventual pregnancy. For all these reasons it is vitally important to have the updated, complete treatment of the subject that this book addresses.

I. C. Y.

Acknowledgments

Of all who helped me in writing this book, I am most indebted to the Mary Ingraham Bunting Institute of Radcliffe College for awarding me a fellowship during the 1986–1987 academic year. The Institute provided me with time and money, without which the book could not have been written; but equally as important to me was the opportunity to be part of a vital community of women scholars and artists from which my work profited immensely. I am also deeply indebted to Dick Yoder, whose way with words was invaluable in converting my medical jargon into English prose. It is good fortune to have a husband who can not only write, but can also type and do the dishes, all with some degree of serenity.

Among the many medical associates who aided my work in various ways, I would like to thank Dr. Juan M. Taveras, who as chairman of the department of radiology at the Massachusetts General Hospital encouraged my project and arranged for my leave of absence from the hospital. Dr. Deborah Hall generously shared her knowledge of ultrasound and contributed her teaching collection. Dr. Jeffrey Newhouse read the manuscript and offered both encouragement and many helpful suggestions. Drs. Richard Pfister, Nicholas Papanicolaou, and Susan Stafford, my colleagues in the genitourinary section at the Massachusetts General Hospital, carried the burden of work there during the year of my absence. Also, I owe a great, trans-Atlantic debt to Dr. Henri Tristant in Paris, who sent me an abundant supply of films permitting the illustration of cases relatively rare in the United States, such as the tumors and tuberculosis of the fallopian tube.

I am very grateful to Edith Tagrin who drew the illustrations for this book. She is a superb artist and a real perfectionist, and her work inspired me to strive for the kind of precision she achieves. I owe great thanks, too, to Ann Bruno who transcribed the entire manuscript and its many revisions into the computer, and always with good humor. Finally, I want to thank my editors at Little, Brown and Company, Susan Pioli and June Goldstein, for their sound advice and the generous amount of time they gave to bringing my work to publication.

This book is dedicated to my parents who, long before I was aware of it, instilled in me the desire to learn and to undertake a professional career. They have continued to support me in every way and at every step, and I now have the pleasure of thanking them with this acknowledgment.

Hysterosalpingography and Pelvic Ultrasound
Imaging in Infertility and Gynecology

Chapter 1
Techniques, Normal Anatomy, and Complications

Hyster = Uterus
Salpinx = Trumpet
Graphein = To write

Hysterosalpingography is the radiographic delineation of the uterus and fallopian tubes. Contrast material introduced into the uterus through the cervical os outlines the inner cavity of the uterus, depicts the lumen of the fallopian tubes, and determines the patency of the tubes. The procedure is monitored by fluoroscopy, and the images are recorded on spot film radiographs.

Indications

Hysterosalpingography is most commonly used in the diagnostic evaluation of infertility. The study is also very helpful in the diagnosis and treatment planning of many gynecologic problems such as abnormal uterine bleeding, intrauterine adhesions, congenital anomalies, and diethylstilbestrol (DES) exposure in utero. It is always recommended prior to special gynecologic surgery such as myomectomy and tubal reconstruction. The hysterosalpingogram is less frequently used but also valuable in the postoperative assessment of uterine and tubal integrity and in tumor staging for endometrial carcinoma (Table 1-1).

Although the hysterosalpingogram has been advocated as a therapeutic technique, it is best regarded as a purely diagnostic procedure that allows the clinician to estimate realistically the chances that pregnancy will occur and the need for surgical intervention. The accurate interpretation of the hysterosalpingogram is greatly enhanced by the frequent correlation with laparoscopy and pelvic ultrasound, which provide complementary views of the female genital tract.

Table 1-1. Indications for hysterosalpingography

Infertility
Congenital abnormality of the uterus
Intrauterine adhesions (Asherman's syndrome)
Prior to myomectomy
Abnormal uterine bleeding
Tubal surgery (pre- and postoperative)
Location of an intrauterine device (after ultrasound)
Diethylstilbestrol exposure in utero
Tumor staging of endometrial carcinoma

Table 1-2. Diagnostic tests used in evaluation of infertility

Semen analysis
Basal body temperature chart
Postcoital test
Endometrial biopsy
Ultrasound of pelvis
Hysterosalpingography
Laparoscopy

Infertility Investigation

The investigation of infertility systematically examines the male and female factors that may contribute to the couple's inability to conceive [13, 27]. Table 1-2 outlines the sequence of tests commonly used to establish the etiology of infertility. The semen analysis and postcoital test evaluate the male factor. These tests provide a count of the total number of sperm, assess their morphology and motility, and assess the ability of the sperm to survive in cervical fluid. The postcoital test also examines the cervical mucus at the time of ovulation when it should be copious and watery. The remaining tests evaluate solely the female factor. The basal body temperature chart and the endometrial biopsy establish the occurrence of normal ovulation. The pelvic ultrasound gives an excellent view of the ovaries and uterus (Fig. 1-1) without radiation exposure or the use of invasive procedures. The hysterosalpingogram outlines the uterine cavity and fallopian tubes (Fig. 1-2) and alerts the endoscopist to the likelihood of any mechanical problems. Diagnostic laparoscopy allows direct observation of the pelvic organs and examines the peritoneum for the presence of adhesions and endometriosis. Laparoscopy includes uterine infusion of methylene blue or indigo carmine dye to assess tubal patency.

Fig. 1-1. Normal pelvic ultrasound. A. Transverse view shows midline uterus and an ovary on each side.

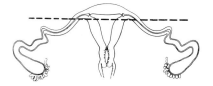

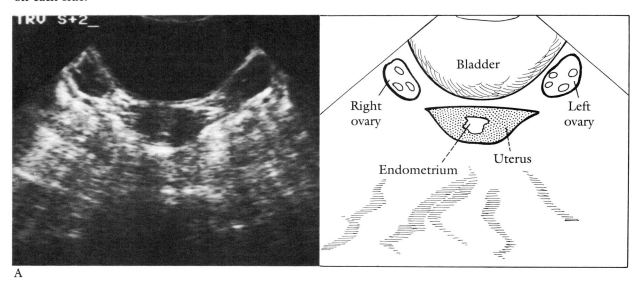

A

B. Sagittal view shows pear-shaped uterus, cervix, and vagina. The endometrial cavity is an oval echo-dense area surrounded by a lucent halo of inner myometrium.

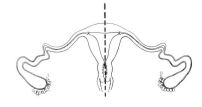

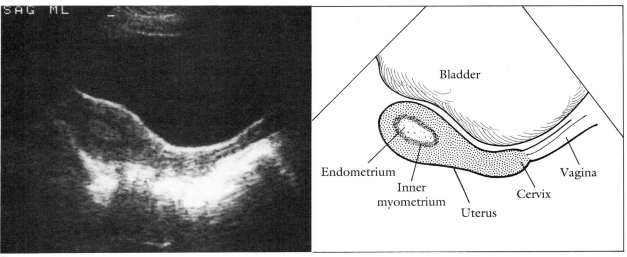

B

4   Techniques, normal anatomy, and complications

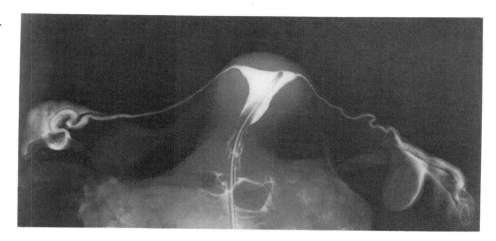

Fig. 1-2. Contrast injection of a normal uterus and fallopian tubes obtained from the 18-year-old victim of an automobile accident.

Techniques

Hysterosalpingograms are often performed by using a tenaculum to grasp the cervix and inserting a rigid obturator into the cervical os to deliver the contrast medium. The application of the sharp tenaculum and traction on the cervix cause pain and cervical bleeding. In many radiology departments the tenaculum has been replaced by a vacuum cannula assembly (Malstrom-Thoren, Göteborg, Sweden). A plastic vacuum cup adheres to the cervix by means of suction and holds the central cannula in the cervical os for injection. The vacuum causes less cervical trauma than the tenaculum, but the rigid obturator within the cervix is a source of pain. The entire assembly is bulky and easily dislodged when the patient moves. The attachment of metal instruments to the cervix and within the vagina, which is required by both the tenaculum and vacuum techniques, causes the patient constant discomfort and hinders her mobility during the procedure.

The use of an 8 Fr Foley balloon catheter for hysterosalpingography circumvents many of the difficulties resulting from the methods mentioned above [28]. The soft rubber Foley catheter slips easily into the cervical os and causes minimal discomfort as the balloon is inflated within the cervical canal. The catheter is self-retaining and no tenaculum or other metal instrument is attached to the cervix or left within the vagina. As a result the patient is comfortable and can move freely during the radiographic study.

Recently several other balloon catheters have become available for hysterosalpingography. They include a 5 Fr polyethylene catheter (Electro-Catheter Corporation, Rahway, New Jersey), a 5 or 7 Fr polyvinylchloride catheter (Akrad Laboratories, Stow, Massachusetts), and a 6.8 Fr polyvinylchloride catheter (Cook, Bloomington, Indiana). The Cook catheter has an end-hole [18], while all the other balloon catheters have a closed end and several side holes. These stiff small caliber catheters are useful but they are not as versatile as the Foley catheter. A soft Foley can be maneuvered into a severely anteverted or retroverted uterus, while an inflexible catheter cannot [1]. In addition, a 10 Fr Foley can serve as a conduit for the introduction of the catheters and wires needed to perform selective salpingography [24]. Selective salpingography is a recently introduced interventional procedure used to deliver contrast directly into the fallopian tube. When the hysterosalpingogram shows interstitial fallopian tube obstruction a 5 Fr polyethylene catheter is inserted through the cut-off end of the Foley catheter and wedged into the tubal ostium. Contrast is then injected to obtain a selective salpingogram. If the fallopian tube fails to fill, a 3 Fr Teflon catheter is advanced directly into the tube over a 0.015-inch platinum-tipped guide wire. The guide wire is removed, and contrast is injected intratubally [24] (see Fig. 2-7).

Procedure

The purpose of the hysterosalpingogram is to obtain as thorough an evaluation of the uterine cavity and fallopian tubes as possible with minimal patient discomfort and minimal radiation exposure. Although it is not usually considered an invasive procedure in the same sense as angiography, the nature of the study entails a considerable invasion of the patient's privacy. By the time the patient leaves the department the examiner will know her menstrual history in detail and will have performed a vaginal examination and catheterization of the uterus. It is therefore very important for the physician to talk to the patient and establish rapport with her before the examination. This interaction should occur before the patient is undressed. If she is already wearing a hospital gown, she should sit on the radiology table or a chair. It is not advisable to initially meet the patient when her legs are already up on stirrups. Such a vulnerable position makes it impossible to develop even the minimum of confidence and trust needed to ensure a successful procedure.

Interview

The preliminary interview serves two purposes. First, it allows the radiologist to obtain an accurate history that includes the reason for the examination, the duration of symptoms, previous pelvic infections or abdominal surgery, contraceptive history, and the date of the last menstrual period. Second, it establishes a personal relationship with the patient during which the physician can give her a realistic and reassuring explanation of the procedure. As a result the patient will be more relaxed, and the hysterosalpingogram is more likely to proceed smoothly.

Preparation

After the initial interview the patient is asked to undress and empty her bladder. The radiology nurse guides her into the x-ray room, helps her into the stirrups, and preps the perineum with a mild soap solution. The nurse's role is invaluable. He or she can answer questions and set the patient at ease by many gestures, including closing the door to assure privacy in a department that is usually bustling with people and activity. The nurse also confirms the date of the last menstrual period and writes it on the requisition, which allows a recheck of menstrual dates since the salpingogram is performed only during the follicular stage of the menstrual cycle. The optimal dates are between the sixth and twelfth days of the cycle, after cessation of menses and before ovulation occurs.

Catheter Insertion

Once the patient is in the lithotomy position the examiner performs a gentle vaginal examination. There is no need for vigorous palpation since the sole purpose of the examination is to determine the position of the cervix and uterus. It is important to note also anteflexion or retroflexion of the uterine body and the presence of any obvious large masses in the pelvis. Subsequently the physician introduces a speculum into the vagina, exposes the cervix, and inserts an 8 Fr Foley catheter into the external cervical os with a long forceps. Table 1-3 lists the basic equipment necessary to perform the procedure. An 8 Fr Foley catheter with a 3-ml balloon is fitted in succession to a Colby adaptor, an extension tube, a two-way stopcock and a 12-ml syringe filled with water soluble contrast medium (Fig. 1-3). The Foley catheter is flushed with contrast to expel the air in its lumen. The long forceps holds the Foley catheter just below the deflated 3-ml balloon. In a single smooth motion the catheter is introduced into the cervical os until the tips of the forceps are against the cervical canal and cannot be advanced. At this point the entire balloon is within the external os and it is slowly inflated with 1 to 3 ml of sterile water. It is essential to continue to grasp the catheter with forceps while the balloon is inflated or the balloon will inevitably "pop out."

The amount of water needed to hold the balloon in place is variable, and with experience the pressure exerted by the thumb on the plunger of the 3 ml syringe will give the operator an idea of how tightly the balloon is wedged within the endocervical canal. The patient should be warned that she will feel some pressure or a crampy sensation while the balloon is being inflated, but this sensation usually abates rapidly after inflation is completed.

Positioning and inflating the Foley balloon can be the most frustrating part of the hysterosalpingogram. Patience is required especially when the

Table 1-3. Equipment needed to perform hysterosalpingogram

8 Fr Foley catheter
Speculum
Long forceps
Colby adaptor
Two-way stopcock
Extension tube
12-ml syringe filled with contrast
3-ml syringe filled with sterile water

Fig. 1-3. Balloon cathe-
ter technique used in
hysterosalpingography.

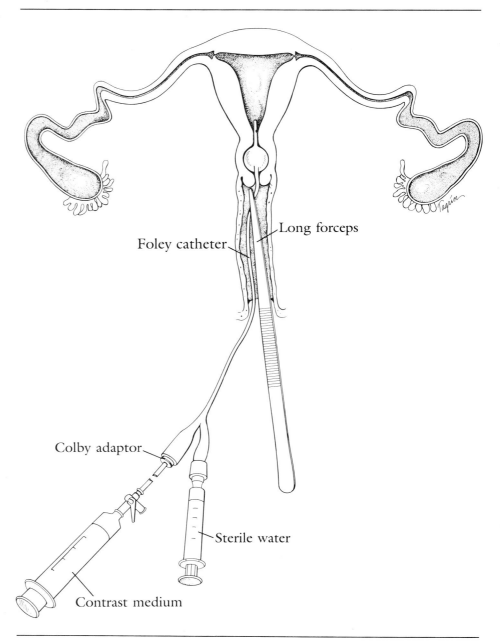

Long forceps

Foley catheter

Colby adaptor

Sterile water

Contrast medium

balloon is extruded repeatedly. Ideally the balloon should be positioned
between the internal and external os (Fig. 1-4); however, if this ideal
cannot be attained, a very satisfactory examination can also be obtained by
threading the catheter farther into the uterine cavity and inflating the balloon within the fundus. Subsequent traction on the catheter will tam-
ponade the balloon against the lower uterine segment and prevent escape of
contrast into the vagina (Fig. 1-5). When gentle traction on the catheter
confirms that it cannot be dislodged from the uterus, the speculum is
removed carefully from the vagina.

Fig. 1-4. Normal hysterosalpingogram. Foley balloon inflated within endocervical canal between the internal os (*solid arrow*) and the external os (*open arrow*). Note free intraperitoneal spill with accumulation of contrast in the cul-de-sac (*CS*).

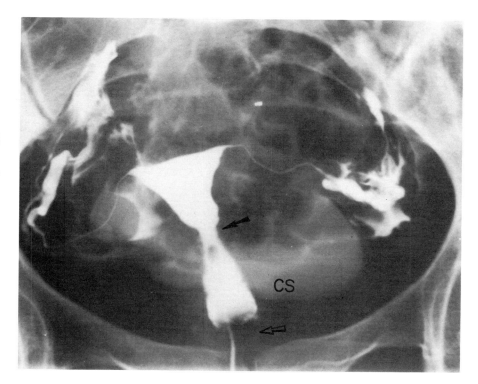

Fig. 1-5. Foley balloon within lower uterine segment (*arrow*). This is a satisfactory hysterosalpingogram although internal os and cervical canal are not demonstrated.

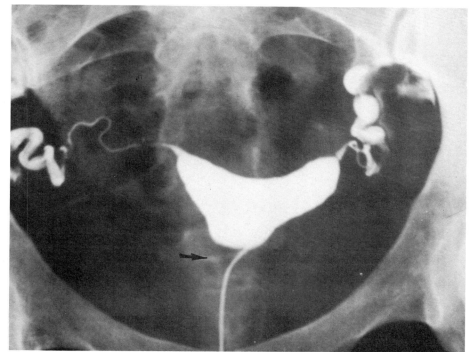

Fig. 1-6. A. Early filling view of uterine cavity shows small submucosal fibroid (*arrows*). B. Further filling and fibroid is completely obscured by contrast.

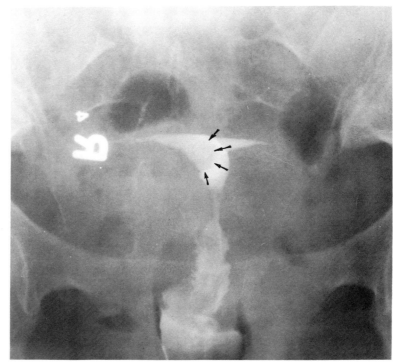

A

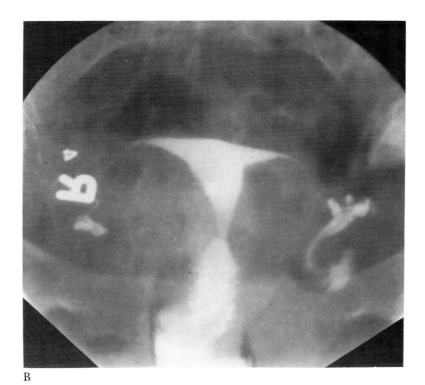

B

Fluoroscopy

At this point the patient is ready for fluoroscopy; her legs are extricated from the stirrups and she is pulled back onto the middle of the radiographic table. The entire examination is recorded on spot films and monitored with the television image intensifier. A preliminary spot film of the pelvis is obtained. Although there are arguments against the need for a preliminary film, it is always wise to obtain one prior to the introduction of contrast medium anywhere in the body. The radiologist infuses the contrast material slowly into the uterus under intermittent fluoroscopic observation and takes the appropriate spot film radiographs. A slow, constant injection prevents the pain caused by sudden distension of the uterus and allows the examiner time to obtain all the images needed. The number of spot films varies but must include (1) an underfilled view of the uterus to detect small endometrial lesions (Fig. 1-6); (2) early filled views of both fallopian tubes before detail is obscured by contrast in the peritoneum; (3) well-filled views of the entire genital tract; and (4) demonstration of ample spill of contrast on both sides.

Films

Usually four or five spot films are sufficient to delineate the anatomy. Most of the films are done in the anteroposterior (AP) projection, but oblique films are often very useful for better display of superimposed or foreshortened structures. A 10- to 20-minute postdrainage film is sometimes needed, especially when intraperitoneal spill of contrast is questionable (Fig. 1-7). Lateral films are seldom used, and because of the large amount of radiation they deliver they are reserved for particularly difficult cases. Some physicians advocate prone films to fill a recalcitrant tube [22] and prone drainage films for better dispersion of contrast. Although rarely used, these views may be useful and are worth consideration.

Fig. 1-7. A. Contrast-filled view of the hysterosalpingogram shows a prominent left fallopian tube containing an air bubble. The right fallopian tube is normal and there appears to be right-sided free intraperitoneal spill of contrast (*arrow*).
B. Drainage view shows bilateral paratubal collections (*arrows*) and minimal free intraperitoneal spill. Laparoscopy showed advanced pelvic endometriosis and extensive adnexal adhesions. (V = vagina.)

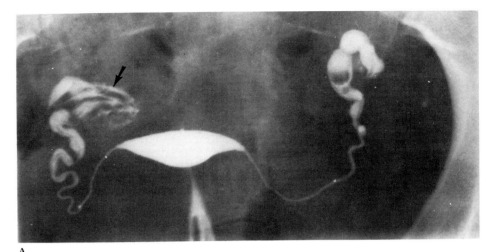

A

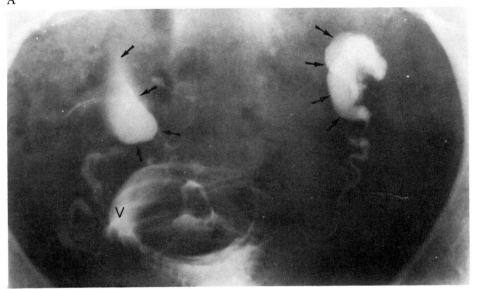

B

Volume of Contrast

The volume of contrast introduced may be as little as 6 ml in a normal study to as much as 60 ml or more in a uterus enlarged by a huge submucous fibroid. Low to moderate pressure can be used to introduce the contrast into the uterus. If the pressure is increased inordinately one of two things may happen: either the patient cries out in pain and demands the study be terminated, or the balloon is expelled out of the uterus into the vagina. Both of these situations should be avoided. At any time when the introduction of contrast is only possible by exerting high pressure, the examiner should turn the stopcock to the off position and wait for the pressure to subside. If the stopcock is not turned off and the syringe is released, the contrast in the uterus rapidly empties into the syringe and has to be rein-

12   Techniques, normal anatomy, and complications

Fig. 1-11. Three normal uterine cavities. A. Prominent fundus with widely separate and rounded uterine horns. B. Moderately prominent fundus. The uterine horns are closer together and are sharper in outline. The internal cervical os (*arrows*) is well demarcated and the cervical canal has serrated walls.

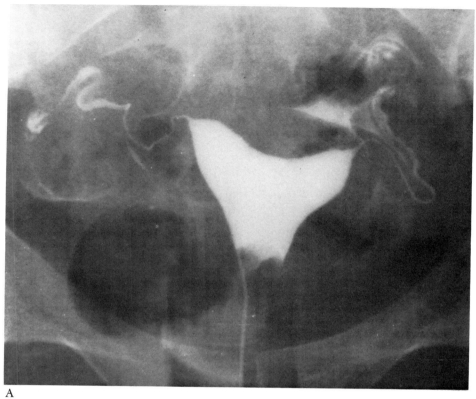

A

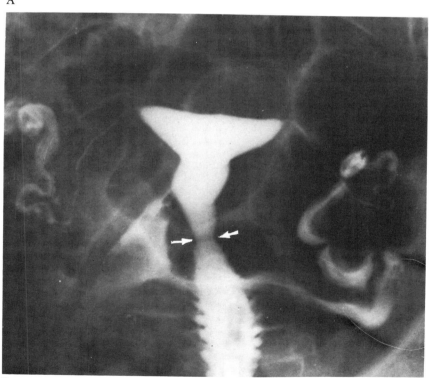

B

Fig. 1-11 (cont.) C. Triangular fundus with inconspicuous uterine horns. Smooth cervical canal and no obvious internal os narrowing.

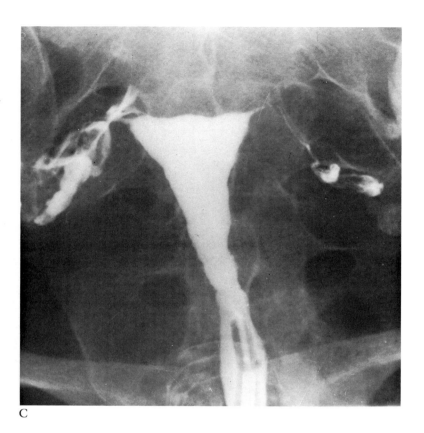

C

Normal Anatomy

The normal uterine cavity is triangular in shape. The base is at the fundus and the apex is inferior and extends into an elongated endocervical canal. Within this format there is as much diversity in the size and shape of the uterine cavity as there is in people's noses; no two are quite the same. The fundus may be elongated with prominent rounded cornua, or short with sharp cornua; the body may taper gradually or abruptly into the endocervix; the cervical canal may be wide or narrow with smooth or serrated walls (Fig. 1-11). The internal os, the junction between the uterine body and cervical canal, is often well-demarcated but is sometimes impossible to locate exactly. Normally the uterus is anteverted over the bladder, and the uterine body is anteflexed in relation to the cervix (Fig. 1-12). Because of the anterior flexion, the image of the fundus often projects over the lower body or cervical canal in the AP view. Oblique views will differentiate the common anteflexed uterus from the much less common retroflexed uterus.

The fallopian tubes arise from the uterine cornua and are divided anatomically into four parts, proceeding laterally: the interstitial segment, isthmus, ampulla, and infundibulum (Fig. 1-13). A thin circumferential lucency at the cornu is not a sphincter but simply a mucosal fold demarcating the transition from endometrium to endosalpinx. Lateral to this fold is the short interstitial or intramural portion of the tube lying within the

18   Techniques, normal anatomy, and complications

Fig. 1-12. Normal ante-
verted and anteflexed
uterus.

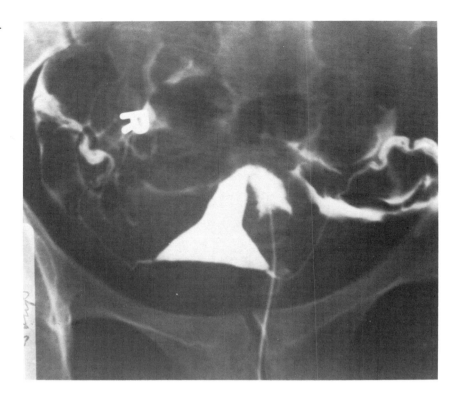

Fig. 1-13. Normal
uterine and tubal
anatomy as delineated
by the hysterosalpingo-
gram.

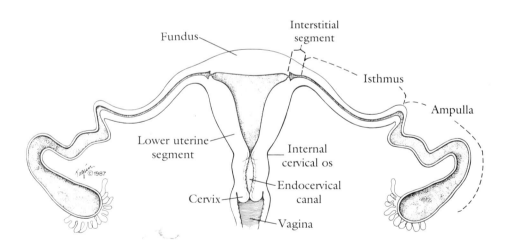

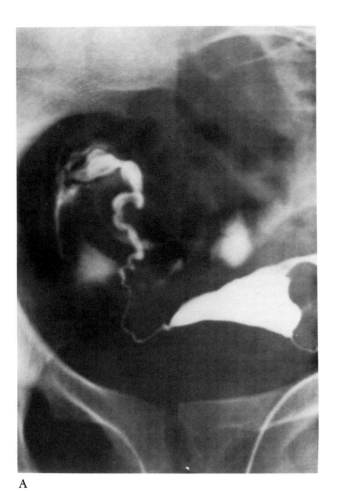 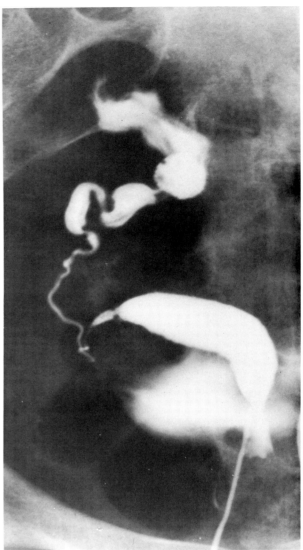

A   B

Fig. 1-14. Two normal
right fallopian tubes.
A. Ampulla is only
mildly prominent. B. Am-
pulla moderately full.
Note normal ampullary
mucosal folds.

Fig. 1-15. Diagrammatic cross-sections of the fallopian tube at (A) interstitial, (B) isthmic, and (C) ampullary regions. The interstitial and isthmic portions of the tube have a thick muscular wall and narrow lumen, while the ampulla has a thin muscular wall and a wide lumen replete with mucosal folds.

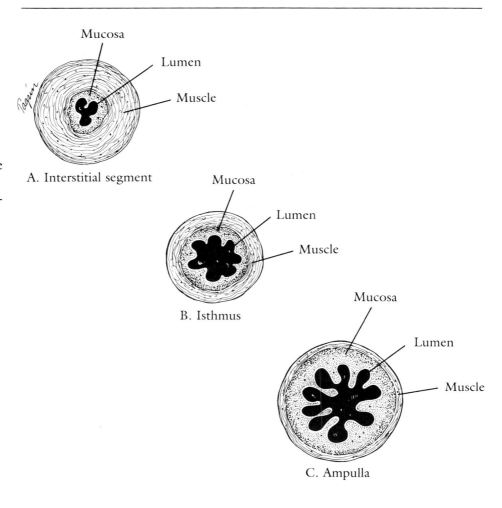

A. Interstitial segment

B. Isthmus

C. Ampulla

myometrium. Next is the long narrow isthmus, which gradually flares into the wide tortuous ampulla (Fig. 1-14). The isthmus has a thick muscular wall and narrow lumen; the ampulla has a thin distensible wall and a wide lumen with prominent mucosal folds (Fig. 1-15). The thin wall allows the marked characteristic swelling of the ampulla referred to as a *hydrosalpinx*. The infundibulum consists of a series of fimbriae or fingers, which radiate around the tubal ostium but are not demonstrated by contrast. Since the fallopian tubes curve posterolaterally, contrast exiting from the tubes tends to accumulate posteriorly in the cul-de-sac. Free intraperitoneal contrast diffuses around bowel loops making it impossible to identify the ovaries.

Fig. 1-16. Same patient as in Fig. 1-6. Hysterosalpingogram shows submucosal myoma along right uterine wall and a left hydrosalpinx (*H*). The right fallopian tube is not filled with contrast because an insufficiently inflated Foley balloon (*arrow*) permits backflow of contrast into vagina (*V*). Bilateral hydrosalpinx was diagnosed at laparoscopy.

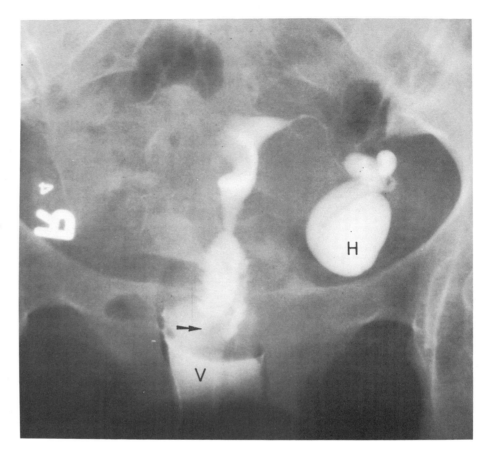

Errors

The most common technical errors incurred during hysterosalpingography include reflux of contrast into the vagina and use of insufficient volume of contrast. Incomplete occlusion of the cervical canal causes contrast to leak into the vagina and can prevent adequate filling of the tubes (Fig. 1-16). Contrast in the vagina may also obscure pelvic pathology. Four to five ml of contrast is often sufficient to outline the internal cavity of the uterus and tubes; however, a much larger volume may be necessary to unequivocally demonstrate tubal patency and free intraperitoneal flow and dispersion (Fig. 1-17).

Fig. 1-17. A. Normal hysterosalpingogram after infusion of 4 ml of contrast. B. Left hydrosalpinx (*H*) and left paratubal adhesions demonstrated after infusion of 8 ml of contrast.

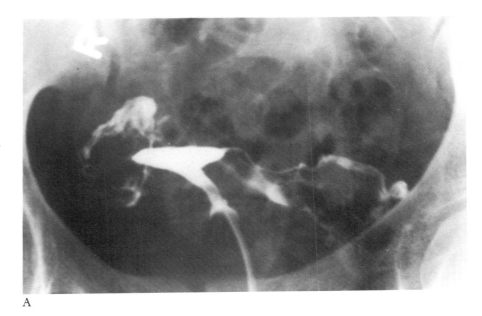

A

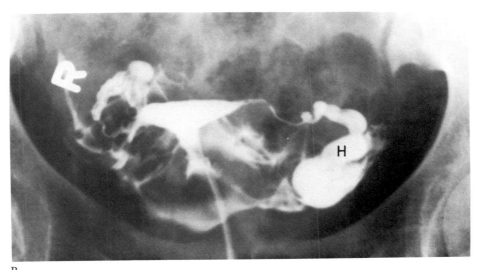

B

Contrasts

Although early hysterosalpingograms were performed with oil soluble contrast medium (Lipiodol was used originally and has been replaced by Ethiodol), the use of oil soluble contrast in hysterosalpingography is an anachronism and should be discontinued. Water soluble contrast medium is the only contrast that can be safely recommended and it would have replaced Ethiodol long ago if it were not for the persistent unfounded belief in the therapeutic effect of oil soluble contrast [21]. Currently Sinografin (meglumine diatrizoate, meglumine iodipamide, and 38% iodine, Squibb) is the most widely used water soluble contrast, but any of the contrast media used for intravenous urography is adequate.

Only water soluble contrast medium provides images with the mucosal detail needed to evaluate uterine endometrial lesions and the tubal ampullary mucosal pattern. It flows readily through the tubes without too much infusion pressure; it disperses easily into the peritoneum and around bowel loops; and it accurately delineates tubal dilatations and paratubal adhesions when present. Immediate postdrainage views are easily obtained as needed. Water soluble contrast is resorbed from the peritoneum within a few hours and is unlikely to induce peritoneal reaction and adhesions.

Common urographic contrasts such as Renografin 60 (meglumine diatrizoate, sodium diatrizoate, and 29% iodine, Squibb) are less expensive than Sinografin but not as popular because their greater fluidity may cause them to flow through the tubes so fast that the peritoneum is flooded with contrast, which obscures uterine and tubal images. New low-osmolality contrast agents such as Hexabrix (ioxaglate meglumine, ioxaglate sodium, and 32% iodine, Mallinckrodt) have been shown to be safe and acceptable for hysterosalpingography [4], but their use will remain limited until their cost becomes less exorbitant.

There is a long-standing and largely uncontested assumption that hysterosalpingography promotes pregnancy, and there are many studies claiming that oil soluble contrast promotes a greater number of pregnancies than water soluble contrast [21]. Pregnancy occurs spontaneously in 35 percent of untreated infertile couples [3]. A number of infertile women undergoing hysterosalpingography will become pregnant at short intervals following the study. Can this pregnancy rate be construed as a therapeutic side effect of the hysterosalpingogram? Probably not, but to date there is no large prospective random study that examines this question. Since the only theoretical advantage of oil soluble contrast is highly questionable and its disadvantages are numerous, continued use of Ethiodol is strongly discouraged.

The disadvantages of Ethiodol include dense images without mucosal detail, immiscible oil droplets aggregating in nondiagnostic patterns (Fig. 1-18) and failing to delineate tubal dilatations or paratubal adhesions, and opaque contrast remaining in the pelvis for months or years and leading to granulomata formation. In addition, venous intravasation incurs the risk of pulmonary and retinal oil emboli. Pulmonary oil embolism is potentially fatal, however, no embolic deaths during hysterosalpingography have been recorded in the last 40 years, most likely because examiners stop contrast infusion as soon as intravasation is recognized under fluoroscopy [2]. Venous intravasation of water soluble contrast, on the other hand, produces no untoward effect; the contrast dissipates in the vascular system and is excreted by the kidneys (Figs. 1-19 and 1-20).

In summary, water soluble contrast medium is recommended because of its better diagnostic qualities and slightly decreased deleterious side effects.

Fig. 1-18. Ethiodol hysterosalpingogram. Oil droplets seen (*arrows*) as contrast is not freely dispersed around bowel loops.

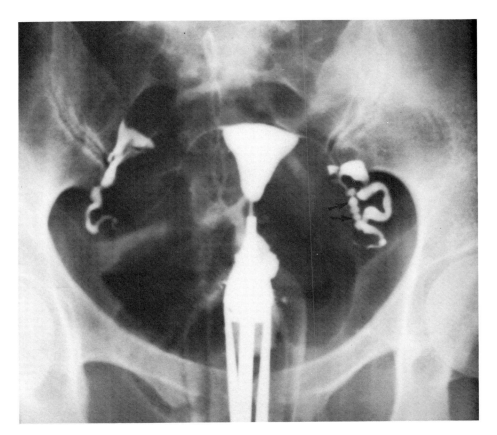

Fig. 1-19. Hysterosalpingogram in a young woman after bilateral tubal ligation. A. Venous intravasation of contrast into the myometrial plexus (*open arrows*) and contrast run-off into the uterine and ovarian veins (*solid arrows*).

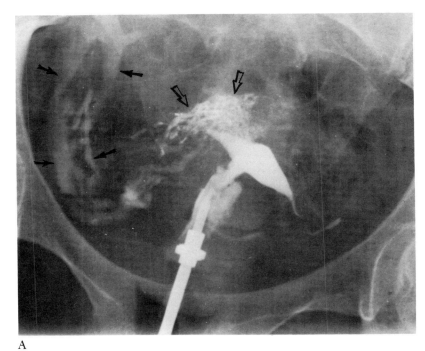

A

Fig. 1-19 (cont.)
B. Abdominal film
shows prompt renal ex-
cretion of contrast (*ar-
rows*). (U = uterus; B
= bladder.)

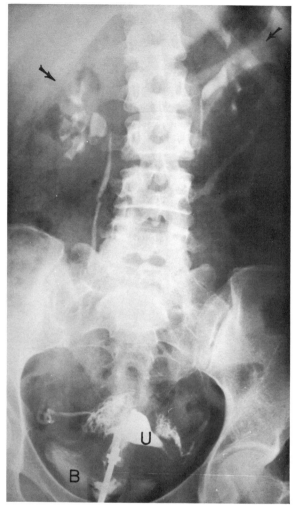

B

Fig. 1-20. Hysterosal-
pingogram performed in
the operating room.
Film of the abdomen
shows extensive intrava-
sation of contrast into
the myometrial, uterine,
and ovarian veins.

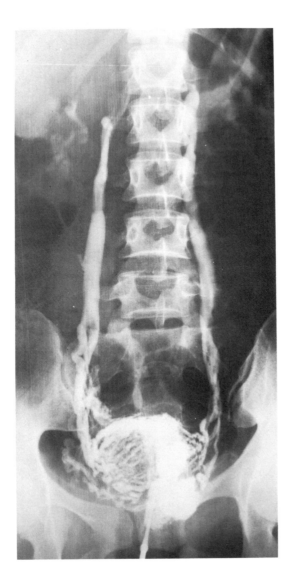

Complications

Pain is the most frequent complication of hysterosalpingography. Other adverse effects include venous and lymphatic intravasation of contrast, acute pelvic infection, radiation exposure, and allergic reactions to contrast (Table 1-5). It has been customary to claim that pain is secondary to peritoneal irritation caused by high-osmolality contrast media; however, recent studies disprove this theory. There is no difference in the amount of pain observed when high-osmolal Sinografin or Renografin is compared with low-osmolal Hexabrix [26]. Use of a tenaculum and obturator, uterine overdistension with contrast, and tubal obstruction contribute to patient pain. It is evident that hysterosalpingography is an uncomfortable procedure since it produces mild to moderate pain in 80 percent of patients and severe pain in up to 4 percent [16]. The pain is usually of brief duration

27

Table 1-5. Complications of hysterosalpingography

Pain
Venous and lymphatic intravasation of contrast
Acute pelvic infection
Radiation exposure
Allergic reaction

and disappears within half an hour after the procedure [12]. Premedication is not routinely advised. Pain will be minimal when the Foley balloon catheter technique is used and contrast is infused slowly. In the presence of tubal obstruction severe pain may be unavoidable and should not be unnecessarily prolonged.

Venous and lymphatic (Fig. 1-21) intravasation of contrast occurs in up to 6 percent of hysterosalpingograms [2]. Predisposing conditions include uterine scarring, tubal obstruction, recent uterine surgery, use of blunt instruments, malplacement of the cannula tip, and excessive injection pressure [19]. Use of larger volumes of contrast does not cause intravasation per se if infusion pressures remain low. Intravasation is innocuous as long as water soluble contrast medium is used.

Pelvic infection is the most serious complication of hysterosalpingography; its incidence ranges from 0.3 to 3.1 percent [25]. Infection is almost exclusively limited to patients with tubal dilatation and a history of previous documented pelvic inflammatory disease. The patient usually presents with pelvic pain and high fever 12 to 48 hours following the study. Cervical cultures are often positive, suggesting that the infection is secondary to the introduction of cervical organisms during the procedure [9]. Prophylaxis with ampicillin or tetracycline has been found ineffective [23]. A recent report recommends that doxycycline be given to all patients showing tubal dilatation [14]. Blanket antibiotic prophylaxis of this kind is costly and treats hundreds of patients unnecessarily; instead patients with tubal dilatation and/or large paratubal accumulations should be advised of their slight increased risk for infection and urged to promptly report any symptoms to their clinicians. The clinician should also be informed of the abnormal findings. When the symptoms appear, vigorous treatment with parenteral antibiotics is indicated to prevent formation of pelvic abscesses. Pelvic ultrasound examination before and during therapy is invaluable to detect formation and evolution of a pelvic collection and to determine the need for surgical drainage (Fig. 1-22).

The radiation dose to the ovaries during hysterosalpingography using standard techniques ranges from 75 to 550 mrad and increases as the number of spot films and the fluoroscopic time increase [17]. These doses are acceptable but can be substantially reduced by using scanning-beam

Fig. 1-21. Hysterosalpingogram in a patient with prior left ectopic pregnancy and left salpingectomy. Lymphatic channels filled with contrast (*arrows*).

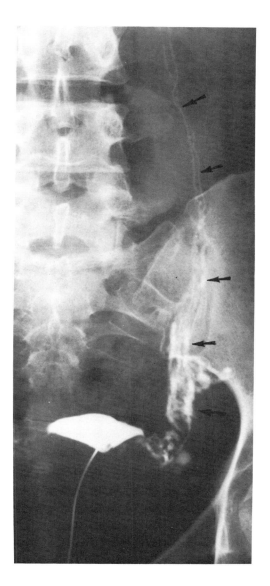

Fig. 1-22. A. Hysterosalpingogram in a patient with several episodes of pelvic infection. A right salpingectomy and a left tuboplasty were performed 1 month prior to the study. There was a moderate left hydrosalpinx and a large left paratubal collection (*arrows*). The patient took doxycycline prophylactically for 3 days. Her temperature rose to 102° F on the day after she stopped the antibiotic. B. Ultrasound on admission (5 days after the hysterosalpingogram) showed a complex left adnexal mass consistent with a tuboovarian abscess. The mass subsided after 2 weeks of intravenous antibiotics.

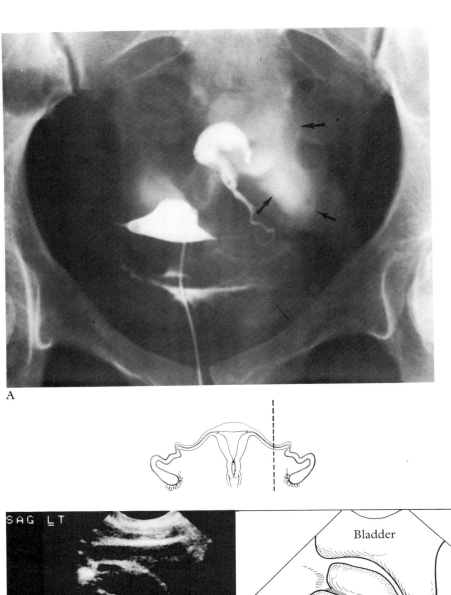

A

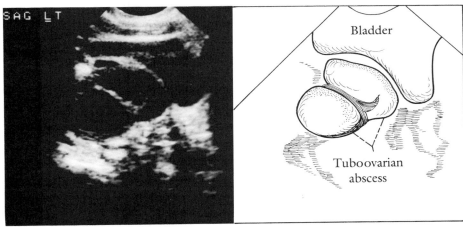

B

Fig. 1-23. Normal digital hysterosalpingogram.

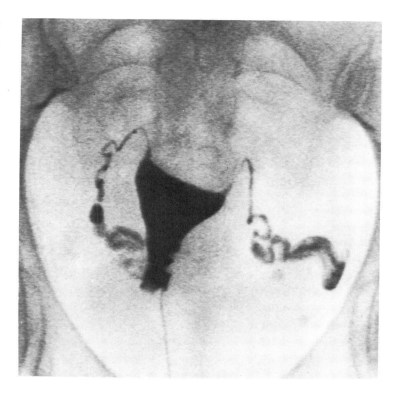

digital radiography where the mean ovarian dose ranges from 2.8 to 7.0 mrad [8]. Although there is some loss of spatial resolution, the digital images are of good diagnostic quality (Fig. 1-23).

Allergic reactions to contrast during hysterosalpingography occur very infrequently and no fatal reactions have ever been reported. Nausea and urticaria occur sometimes after venous intravasation of contrast. Rarely a patient experiences a vasovagal reaction characterized by hypotension and bradycardia, which requires administration of atropine and intravenous fluids. Very seldom a patient suffers excruciating abdominal pain after normal spill of contrast into the peritoneal cavity. This so-called idiosyncratic reaction to contrast can be differentiated from pelvic infection by the absence of fever and is treated symptomatically with analgesics.

Table 1-6. Contraindications to hysterosalpingography

Active uterine bleeding
Acute pelvic infection
Pregnancy

Contraindications

Active uterine bleeding, acute pelvic infection, and pregnancy are contraindications to hysterosalpingography (Table 1-6). Brisk bleeding from a recent dilatation and curettage is an absolute contraindication, but scant bleeding secondary to menses or a submucous fibroid is only a relative contraindication. Contrast infused into the uterus of a patient who has had recent uterine surgery will pass directly into the uterine veins (Fig. 1-24) and will not provide any diagnostic information. Contrast infused into the uterus of a menstruating patient will successfully outline the uterus and tubes, but blood clots in the uterine cavity may interfere with the diagnosis of small filling defects.

Acute pelvic infection is an absolute contraindication to a contrast study of the uterus. Vaginal infections, however, are very common and allow the continuation of the study following cleansing of the cervix and vagina as needed to remove excessive exudate.

Uterine manipulation during hysterosalpingography will not usually abort an early pregnancy, nor is the amount of radiation delivered proven injurious to the fetus; nevertheless, it is wisest to perform the study when there is no possibility of pregnancy. Patients who have regular menstrual cycles are studied only during the follicular phase of the cycle. Anovulatory patients may need a pregnancy test prior to the study. In spite of all precautions a hysterosalpingogram sometimes discloses an early pregnancy. It is necessary to inform the patient and the clinician of the situation and provide them with an estimate of the radiation dose to the fetus based on the number of spot films and the time of fluoroscopy. This is done primarily for medicolegal reasons, since fetal doses seldom exceed 1 rad and therapeutic abortion is not usually recommended [7].

Fig. 1-24. Hysterosalpingogram attempted 1 day after dilatation and curettage. The contrast does not outline the uterine cavity; instead it goes directly into the myometrial venous plexus and uterine veins.

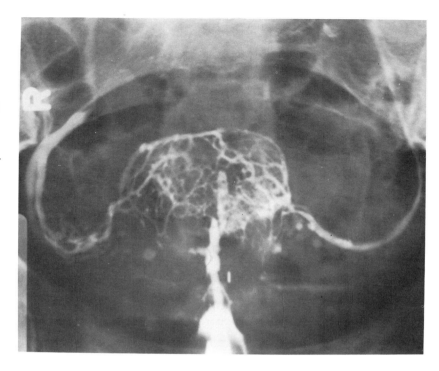

Interpretation

The interpretation of the hysterosalpingogram is dependent on the radiologist's experience as well as a thorough knowledge of (1) the patient's history; (2) normal anatomy and common variants; (3) the examination's strengths and weaknesses as determined by comparison with laparoscopy; and (4) pelvic ultrasound findings when available. It is essential to be completely familiar with the patient's problem. A tubular structure is limited in the way it can react to disease: It can become stenotic or dilated. Tubal dilatation may thus result from infection, endometriosis, or surgery, depending on previous events or symptomatology.

Laparoscopy

Laparoscopy was introduced in the United States in the early 1970s and is used routinely as a diagnostic and therapeutic tool in the evaluation of the female pelvis. Laparoscopy, the study of the external anatomy, complements hysterosalpingography, the study of the luminal anatomy. In the 1980s rates of agreement between the two studies range from 67 to 86 percent [5,6,10,11,15,20] (Table 1-7). There is a higher concordance between the findings at hysterosalpingography and laparoscopy when the former is performed by an experienced radiologist, working in close association with the gynecologist and using water soluble contrast. Hysterosalpingograms average a false-positive rate of 6 to 29 percent and a false-negative rate of 4 to 7 percent [6]. Proximal tubal obstructions caused by

Table 1-7. Correlation between hysterosalpingography and laparoscopy

Author	Agreement (%)
Musich and Behrman (1982)	75
Nordenskjöld and Ahlgren (1983)	71
Holst, Abyholm, and Borgersen (1983)	86
Duff, et al. (1983)	67
Portuondo, et al. (1984)	71
Snowden, Jarrett, and Dawood (1984)	86

apparent spasm or insufficient contrast account for most of the false-positive hysterosalpingograms. Undetected paratubal adhesions are responsible for most of the false-negative studies.

Ultrasound

Pelvic ultrasound provides another diagnostic method for scrutiny of the female pelvis. Its value lies mainly in its ability to outline the ovaries and adnexal regions not visible on hysterosalpingogram. When one images the uterus sonography and hysterosalpingography are complementary studies. Ultrasound can suggest the presence of a uterine fibroid, and hysterosalpingography can demonstrate its submucous location. Similarly ultrasound can show the presence of a congenital uterine duplication, and hysterosalpingography can delineate its exact internal configuration.

References

1. Austin, R. M., et al. Catheter hysterosalpingography. *Radiology* 151:249, 1984.
2. Bateman, B. G., Nunley, W. C., and Kitchin, J. D. Intravasation during hysterosalpingography using oil-based contrast media. *Fertil. Steril.* 34:439, 1980.
3. Collins, J. A., et al. Treatment-independent pregnancy among infertile couples. *N. Engl. J. Med.* 309:1201, 1983.
4. Davies, A. C., et al. The use of a low-osmolality contrast medium in hysterosalpingography: comparison with a conventional contrast medium. *Clin. Radiol.* 36:533, 1985.
5. Duff, D. E., et al. Hysterosalpingography and laparoscopy: a comparative study. *AJR* 141:761, 1983.
6. Holst, N., Abyholm, T., and Borgersen, A. Hysterosalpingography in the evaluation of infertility. *Acta Radiol. [Diagn.] (Stockh.)* 24:253, 1983.
7. Jacobson, A., and Conley, J. G. Estimation of fetal dose to patients undergoing diagnostic x-ray procedures. *Radiology* 120:683, 1976.
8. Kushner, D. C., et al. Radiation dose reduction during hysterosalpingography: an application of scanning-beam digital radiography. *Radiology* 161:31, 1986.

9. Moller, B. R., et al. Pelvic inflammatory disease after hysterosalpingography associated with *Chlamydia trachomatis* and *Mycoplasma hominis*. *Br. J. Obstet. Gynaecol.* 91:1181, 1984.

10. Musich, J. R., and Behrman, S. J. Infertility laparoscopy in perspective: review of five hundred cases. *Am. J. Obstet. Gynecol.* 143:293, 1982.

11. Nordenskjöld, F., and Ahlgren, M. Laparoscopy in female infertility. Diagnosis and prognosis for subsequent pregnancy. *Acta Obstet. Gynecol. Scand.* 62:609, 1983.

12. Owens, O. M., et al. Reduction of pain following hysterosalpingography by prior analgesic administration. *Fertil. Steril.* 43:146, 1985.

13. Patton, G. W., and Kistner, R. W. *Atlas of Infertility Surgery* (2nd ed.). Boston: Little, Brown, 1984. Pp. 3–19.

14. Pittaway, D. E., et al. Prevention of acute pelvic inflammatory disease after hysterosalpingography: efficacy of doxycycline prophylaxis. *Am. J. Obstet. Gynecol.* 15:623, 1983.

15. Portuondo, J. A., et al. Clinical selection of infertile patients for laparoscopy. *Int. J. Fertil.* 29:234, 1984.

16. San Fillippo, J. S., Yussman, M. A., and Smith, D. Hysterosalpingography in the evaluation of infertility: a six year review. *Fertil. Steril.* 30:636, 1978.

17. Sheikh, H. H., and Yussman, M. A. Radiation exposure of ovaries during hysterosalpingography. *Am. J. Obstet. Gynecol.* 124:307, 1976.

18. Sholkoff, S. D. Balloon hysterosalpingography catheter. *AJR* 149:995, 1987.

19. Siegler, A. M. Hysterosalpingography. *Fertil. Steril.* 40:139, 1983.

20. Snowden, E. V., Jarrett, J. C., and Dawood, M. Y. Comparison of diagnostic accuracy of laparoscopy, hysteroscopy, and hysterosalpingography in evaluation of female infertility. *Fertil. Steril.* 41:709, 1984.

21. Soules, M. R., and Spadoni, L. R. Oil versus aqueous media for hysterosalpingography: a continuing debate based on many opinions and few facts. *Fertil. Steril.* 38:1, 1982.

22. Spring, D. B., and Boll, D. A. Prone hysterosalpingography. *Radiology* 136:235, 1980.

23. Stumpf, P. G., and March, C. M. Febrile morbidity following hysterosalpingography: identification of risk factors and recommendations for prophylaxis. *Fertil. Steril.* 33:487, 1980.

24. Thurmond, A. S., et al. Fallopian tube obstruction: selective salpingography and recanalization. *Radiology* 163:511, 1987.

25. Tuveng, J. M., et al. Hysterosalpingography: value in estimating tubal function and risk of infectious complications. *Acta Eur. Fertil.* 16:125, 1985.

26. Winfield, A. C., et al. Hexabrix as a contrast agent for hysterosalpingography. *Radiology* 34:439, 1980.

27. Winfield, A. C., and Wentz, A. C. *Diagnostic Imaging of Infertility*. Baltimore: Williams & Wilkins, 1987. Pp. 1–8.

28. Yoder, I. C., and Pfister, R. C. Balloon catheter hysterosalpinography. *AJR* 133:335, 1979.

29. Yoder, I. C., and Pfister, R. C. Angiodilator technique for hysterosalpingography in cervical os stenosis. *Radiology* 139:228, 1981.

Chapter 2
Diseases of the Fallopian Tube

Since the seminal duct from its beginning to its end has a likeness of the bent-parts of this classic instrument, separate or attached, therefore, it has been called by me the Uteri Tuba.

Gabriel Fallopius (1523–1562)

Infertility, defined as 1 year of unprotected intercourse without conception, affects approximately 15 percent of couples in the United States. The woman is infertile in 50 percent of couples, the male is responsible in 30 to 40 percent of cases, and no cause is found in 10 to 20 percent of couples [17]. Causes of female infertility include hormonal disturbances, cervical mucus disorders, and, most frequently, tubal occlusions. As an increasing number of women postpone childbearing into their thirties, they experience an increased risk of intercurrent tubal disease and tubal obstruction resulting in infertility. Venereal infection, pelvic infection associated with intrauterine devices or therapeutic abortion, endometriosis, and pelvic surgery are the leading causes of tubal scarring and peritoneal adhesions. The hysterosalpingogram is an integral part of infertility evaluation and of particular importance in the diagnosis of fallopian tube pathology because it is the only diagnostic procedure that allows unequivocal demonstration of internal tubal anatomy. Tubal obstruction and dilatation is demonstrated in 24 to 50 percent of hysterosalpingograms. The most common cause of tubal abnormality is previous pelvic infection (Table 2-1).

Pelvic Inflammatory Disease

Pelvic inflammatory disease and acute salpingitis are used interchangeably to indicate infection of the fallopian tubes caused by sexually transmitted microorganisms [43]. The etiology of acute salpingitis varies according to geographic area and time of the study. In the United States gonococcal infections are still common. The organisms cultured in a recent U.S. study of pelvic infection include *Neisseria gonorrhoeae* (40%), *Chlamydia trachomatis* (27%), and mixed aerobic and anaerobic bacteria (46%) [38]. In Scandinavian countries the incidence of gonococcal salpingitis has decreased to 10 percent, while the overall incidence of salpingitis has increased [44]. *C. trachomatis, Mycoplasma hominis, Ureaplasma urealyticum* and anaerobic bacteria are the pathogens increasingly responsible for venereal disease in developed countries. The intrauterine device (IUD) is an important contributing cause to pelvic infection, while oral contraceptive pills appear to offer a protective effect [9]. Tuberculosis, a cause of tubal infection in the past, is now very rare in Western industrialized countries.

N. gonorrhoeae and other sexually transmitted organisms usually colonize the cervix and ascend to the tubes by way of the uterus. There is an initial endometritis and subsequent endosalpingitis. The endometrium is able to

Table 2-1. Common causes of tubal obstruction

Pelvic infection
Tubal ligation
Endometriosis
Adhesions from previous pelvic surgery

Fig. 2-1. A. Transverse ultrasound shows bilateral tuboovarian abscesses. Irregular masses converge in the cul-de-sac. These masses have shaggy walls and a mixed echogenic pattern.

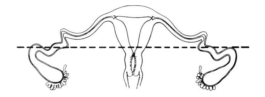

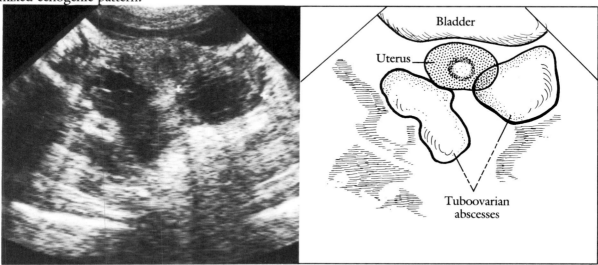

A

B. After 2 weeks of antibiotic therapy a repeat ultrasound demonstrates decrease in size of tuboovarian abscesses. (Courtesy of Dr. Deborah Hall, Boston, Mass.)

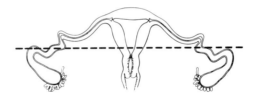

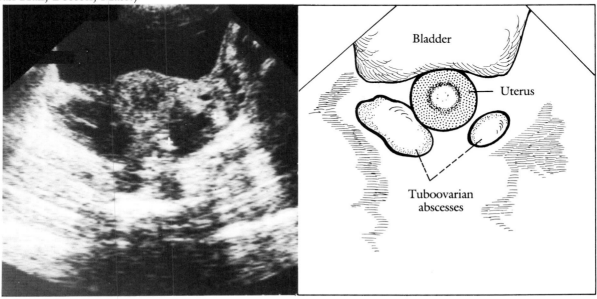

B

renew itself through normal cyclic changes, while the tubal mucosa more easily incurs permanent damage. Partial destruction of tubal cells render the tube more susceptible to repeat pelvic infections. During the acute episode exudate and pus spills through the tubes into the peritoneum leading to peritonitis, tuboovarian abscesses, and cul-de-sac collections. Fimbrial fibrosis and tubal occlusion are common sequelae. Pus can accumulate in an occluded ampulla resulting in a pyosalpinx, which, after antibiotic treatment, becomes a hydrosalpinx and the purulent exudate is replaced by sterile serous fluid.

A review of the effects of treated pelvic infection on infertility revealed tubal occlusion after one infection in 12.8 percent; after two infections in 35.5 percent; and after three or more infections in 75 percent of women [42]. Tubal occlusion is more common after nongonococcal than after gonococcal salpingitis. Women with tubal obstruction have a significantly greater incidence of sterility and ectopic pregnancy than controls.

Ultrasound

In the early phases of acute pelvic infection physical examination is painful to the patient and pelvic sonography helps define the extent of pelvic involvement. The most common sonographic pattern shows a disorganized pelvis filled with solid and cystic areas [37]. The definition between the uterus and adnexal structures is lost secondary to local inflammation. Frequently ultrasound demonstrates single or multiple adnexal and cul-de-sac masses (Fig. 2-1). It is seldom possible to differentiate a pyosalpinx from other pelvic abscesses.

Tuboovarian and pelvic abscesses may be cystic, but more often they contain debris that appears as diffuse internal echoes; rarely they may have septations, a fluid-debris level, or acoustic shadowing secondary to air bubbles [2]. A hypoechoic uterus and loss of endometrial echoes secondary to endometritis is seen infrequently. Most of the findings described previously are nonspecific and may also be seen in postoperative pelvic abscess or hematoma, ovarian cyst or neoplasm, endometriosis, and ruptured ectopic pregnancy. The clinical history and findings are crucial in establishing the diagnosis of pelvic infection and initiating antibiotic therapy. Resolution of pelvic abscesses is easily documented by ultrasound. A patient who has had single or multiple episodes of pelvic infection and who is clinically quiescent but complains of infertility may have an entirely normal-appearing pelvic ultrasound examination [17]. Very occasionally a hydrosalpinx can be demonstrated as a tubular dilatation extending between the uterus and the ovary (Fig. 2-2).

Fig. 2-2. Transverse sonograms in a 37-year-old woman with a history of pelvic inflammatory disease demonstrate: (A) dilated tubular structures on each side of the uterus and

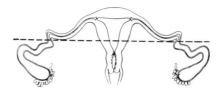

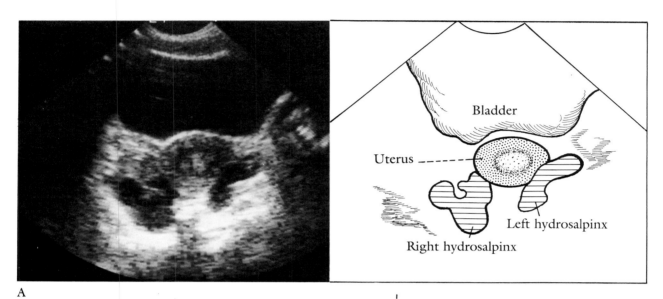

A

(B) good delineation of a dilated left fallopian tube at a higher level.

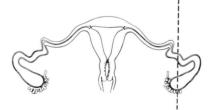

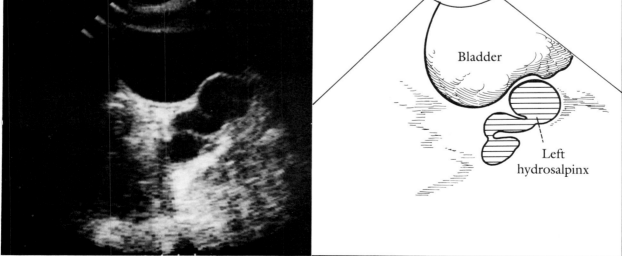

B

Fig. 2-2 (cont.)
C. Hysterosalpingogram
on the same patient
confirms the presence of
bilateral hydrosalpinx
(*H*). Laparoscopy
showed severe ampullary
dilatation on both sides.

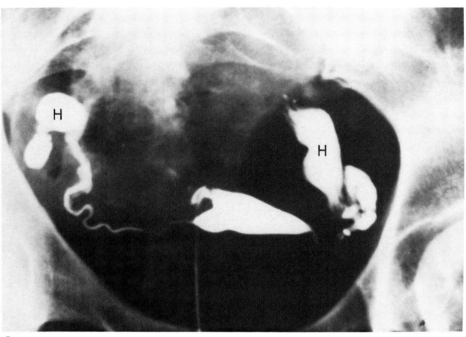

C

Hysterosalpingography

The hysterosalpingogram is performed long after the acute pelvic infection has occurred and when infertility instead has become the main problem. Tubal obstruction may occur at any level. The hysterosalpingogram readily localizes tubal obstruction but, with the possible exception of salpingitis isthmica nodosa, gives no specific information regarding the nature of the pathologic process causing the obstruction. The radiologist offers a differential diagnosis based on the radiologic image; the patient's history, symptoms, and physical findings; and the results of previous ultrasound and laparoscopy.

Interstitial Obstruction. Interstitial or cornual obstruction occurs in 10 to 22 percent [33] of all tubal obstructions demonstrated during hysterosalpingography. It is postulated that true proximal tubal obstruction is more often associated with postpartum or postabortal pelvic infection. The severe endometritis produced occludes the proximal tube and may prevent involvement of the distal tube. Proximal occlusion precludes evaluation of the distal tube and limits availability of diagnostic information.

Tubal spasm, the inability to fill the tube with contrast because of transient muscular spasm of the interstitial segment must be differentiated from true organic obstruction of the proximal fallopian tube.

In past studies tubal spasm was often described as one of the major sources of error in hysterosalpingography. Many drugs, such as atropine, nitroglycerin, sympathomimetic drugs, narcotics, and, more recently, glu-

42   Diseases of the fallopian tube

Fig. 2-3. Hysterosalpin-gogram shows a right cornual obstruction. Contrast outlines the triangular cavity of the interstitial segment of fallopian tube just lateral to mucosal fold (*arrow*).

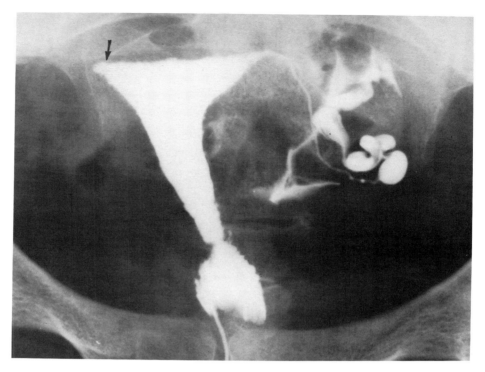

cagon have all been administered in an unsuccessful effort to prevent tubal muscular spasm [46]. These treatments are unsuccessful because tubal spasm stems from multiple factors. Tubal spasm is probably secondary to a combination of patient anxiety, painful techniques, and rapid contrast injection. In a setting where the emphasis is on patient comfort and gentle technique, tubal spasm rarely occurs.

A rounded "breastlike" shape of the uterine horn suggests cornual spasm [19]. In true cornual obstruction the triangular cavity of the interstitial tube is sharply demarcated and the sloping walls of the uterine horn meet at an acute angle, either lateral or proximal to the normal mucosal fold (Fig. 2-3). Occasionally a single fallopian tube fills preferentially with contrast, while the contralateral tube shows apparent interstitial obstruction. Often tubal filling is easily accomplished by allowing a small interval of rest before introducing additional contrast into the uterine cavity (Fig. 2-4). Very rarely the tip of the Foley catheter accidentally occludes the uterotubal junction, and retracting allows tubal filling (Fig. 2-5). When a tube fails to fill, all efforts should be made to fill the empty tube with the help of gravity by turning the patient toward the nonfilling side or placing her prone while introducing more contrast (Fig. 2-6). If after these maneuvers the tube remains occluded, it is likely that a true mechanical cornual obstruction exists.

Fig. 2-4. Hysterosalpingogram performed on a 28-year-old anovulatory patient before she received hormonal ovarian stimulation. A. There was a normal left fallopian tube and an apparent right interstitial obstruction (*arrow*). B. Infusion of additional contrast filled the normal right fallopian tube. Note infantile proportions of the uterus secondary to lack of normal estrogen effect.

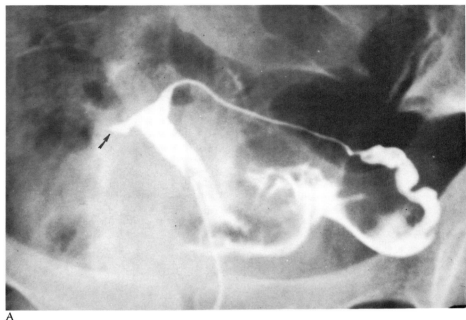

A

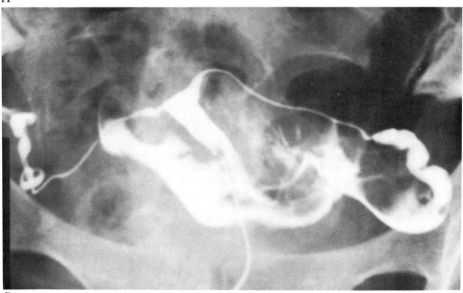

B

Interstitial obstruction may extend into the isthmic segment [11] but seldom involves the ampulla. Selective salpingography can be used to bridge the short cornual occlusion and demonstrate the tube beyond the obstruction [39]. A 0.015-inch platinum-tipped guide wire is introduced into the tubal ostium and manipulated through the occluded area. A 3 Fr Teflon catheter is passed over the guide wire, the wire is removed, and contrast is infused into the isthmic and ampullary segments of the tube.

Fig. 2-5. Hysterosalpin-
gogram obtained on a
26-year-old DES daugh-
ter with primary infertility. A. There was a nor-
mal left fallopian tube.
The Foley balloon cathe-
ter completely filled the
small uterine cavity and
the catheter tip (*arrow*)
effectively occluded the
right tube. B. After the
Foley catheter was
pulled back slightly from
the fundus into the body
of the uterus, additional
contrast infusion filled a
normal right fallopian
tube.

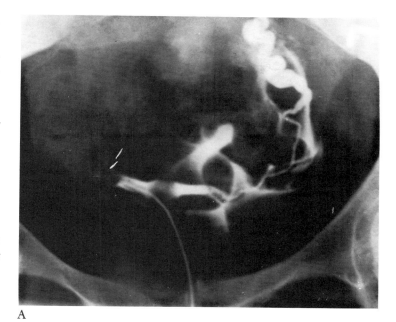

A

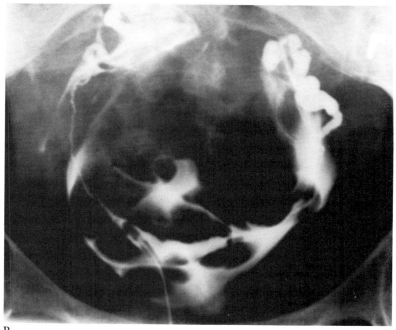

B

Fig. 2-6. A. Hysterosal-
pingogram shows a left
cornual obstruction (*ar-
row*). B. Prone film and
infusion of more con-
trast corroborate pres-
ence of true cornual ob-
struction (*arrow*). At
laparoscopy methylene
blue did not flow into
left fallopian tube. (V =
vagina; CS = cul-de-
sac.)

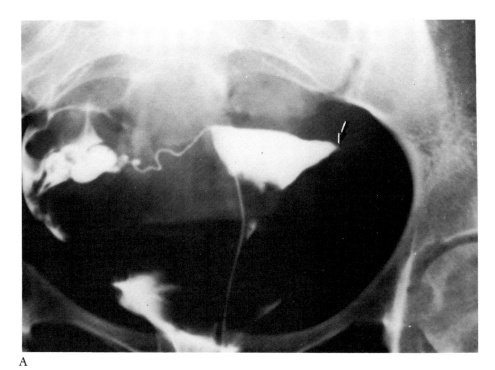

A

B

Fig. 2-7. A. Hysterosal-
pingogram performed in
a 40-year-old woman
with a history of 18
years of IUD use and 1
year of infertility since
the removal of the IUD.
Both cornua are irregu-
lar, and there is bilateral
interstitial occlusion (*arrows*). B and C. Right
and left selective salpingography obtained
through a 3 Fr Teflon
catheter (*arrows*) shows
normal tubes distal to
cornual obstruction and
free intraperitoneal spill.
(CS = cul-de-sac.)

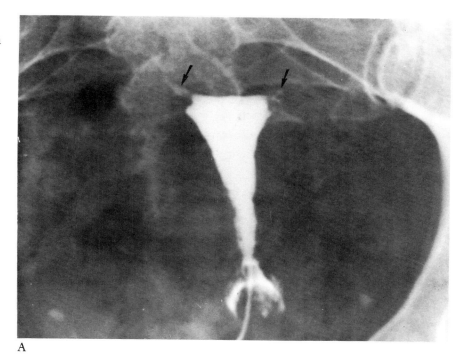

A

B

Fig. 2-7 (cont.)

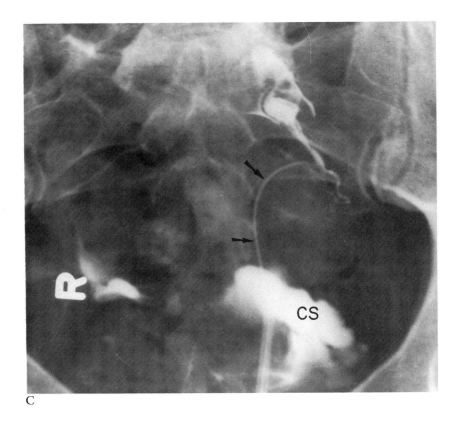

C

This procedure allows evaluation of the fallopian tube beyond the obstructed interstitial segment (Fig. 2-7). The minuscule tunnel forged by the guide wire is likely to reocclude promptly, and it is doubtful that selective salpingography will have any therapeutic value.

The principal causes of cornual obstruction include fibrosis secondary to pelvic infection or tubal ligation, salpingitis isthmica nodosa, intramucosal endometriosis, and chronic tubal inflammation. A strategically located uterine lesion, such as a uterine polyp, a submucous myoma, endometrial adhesions, or a tumor, could obstruct the proximal tube but does so only very rarely. Tubal polyps characteristically occur within the interstitial segment of the fallopian tube but seldom cause obstruction.

Isthmic Obstruction. Isthmic obstruction occurs in 5 to 7 percent of hysterosalpingograms [34] and is secondary to salpingectomy, tubal ligation, infectious scarring, and endometriosis. Obstruction of the narrow, nondistensible isthmic segment appears as an abrupt termination of the tubal lumen several centimeters lateral to the uterine horn. Dilatation of the isthmus is uncommon. A small bulbous clublike swelling may be seen following tubal ligation (Fig. 2-8). Very irregular luminal distension may result from tuberculous salpingitis.

Fig. 2-12. Hysterosalpingogram in a 36-year-old woman with a history of repeated pelvic infection and previous tubal surgery for adhesions. There was bilateral hydrosalpinx with moderate ampullary dilatation and no free intraperitoneal spill. Laparoscopy showed clubbed and dilated ampullae and severe adnexal adhesions. (From I. C. Yoder and J. H. Newhouse. Use of the Foley catheter in hysterosalpingography. *Appl. Radiology* 11:1, 68, 1982. Reprinted with permission.)

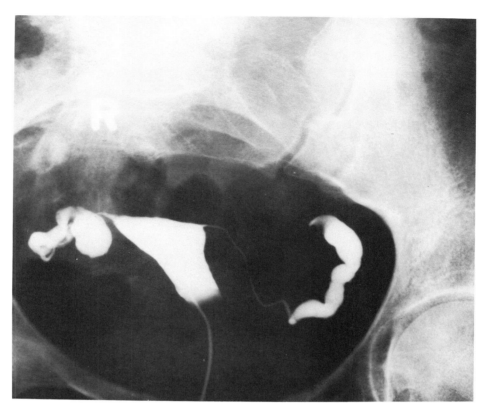

Fig. 2-13. A. Mild bilateral hydrosalpinx, no intraperitoneal spill. Small outpouchings or diverticula surround the left ampulla. B. Detailed view of left ampulla shows ampullary diverticula (*arrows*). Patient had past history of severe pelvic infection with appropriate antibiotic treatment delayed several weeks. Although this "tufted" appearance of the ampulla has been described in tubal tuberculosis, in this case it indicated the severity of the infection and not the etiology since the patient did not have tuberculosis.

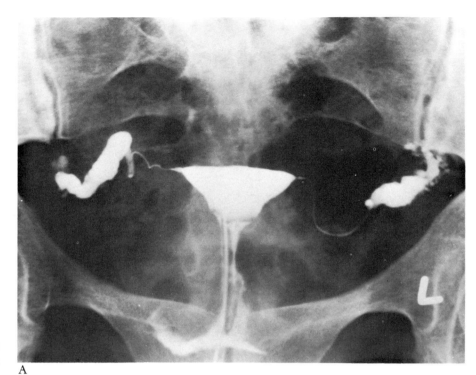

A

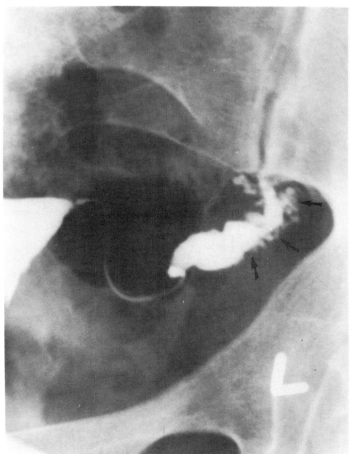

B

Fig. 2-14. A. Mild left hydrosalpinx, no peritoneal spill. Previous right salpingectomy for ectopic pregnancy was performed. B. Drainage film confirms abnormal dilatation and obstruction of the left ampulla.

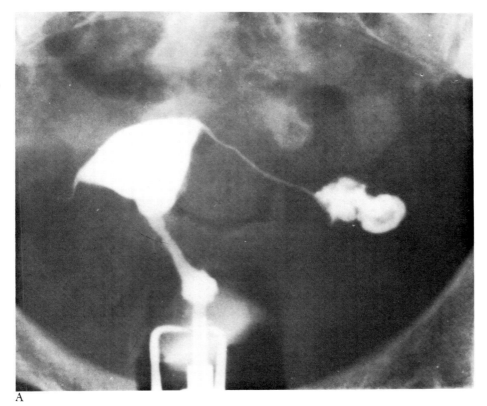

A

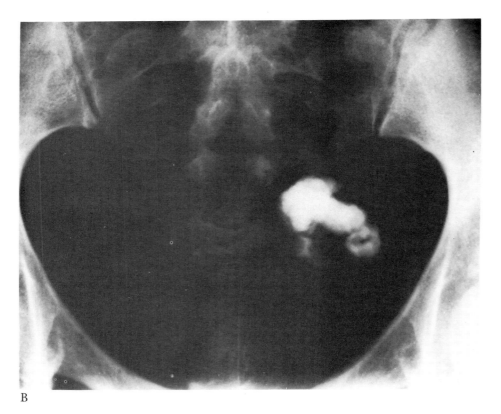

B

Fig. 2-15. Hysterosalpingogram performed with a digital radiographic system on a 33-year-old woman with past history of pelvic inflammatory disease. A. Initial film shows what may be interpreted as free spill into the cul-de-sac (*arrow*) from normal right tube. (From D. C. Kushner, et al., Radiation dose reduction during hysterosalpingography: an application of scanning-digital beam radiography. *Radiology* 161:31–33, 1986. Reprinted with permission.) B. As more contrast is introduced there is no dispersion and a paratubal collection is suspected.

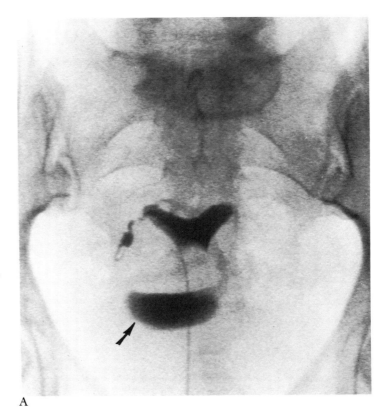

A

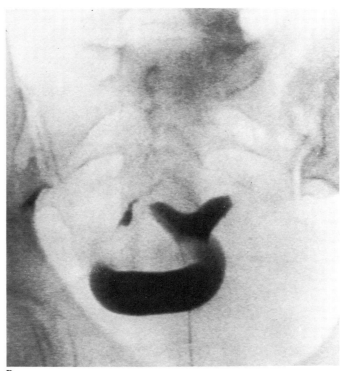

B

Fig. 2-15 (cont.)
C. Drainage film de-
lineates a huge right hy-
drosalpinx. There is also
a left cornual obstruc-
tion. Surgery confirmed
both findings.

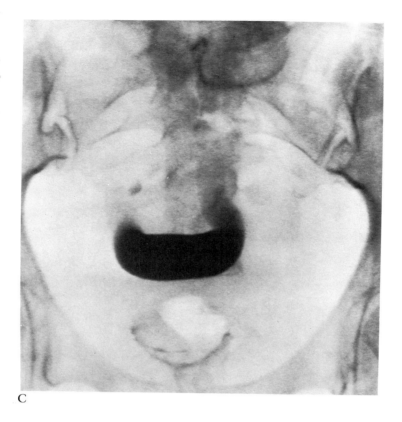

C

of contrast into the vagina. At the other end of the spectrum, a hydrosalpinx may be so severe that what initially seems to be free intraperitoneal
spill proves to be an enormously dilated hydrosalpinx (Fig. 2-15). A delayed upright film may show a fluid-contrast level in the dilated ampulla.
However, the upright view is not necessary if a sufficient volume of contrast
is used to adequately demonstrate the enlarged tube. Sufficient contrast is
especially important if contrast flows preferentially into a dilated tube at the
expense of the other tube, which may be similarly affected. Once the dilated
ampulla(e) are outlined, a supine or prone drainage film is invaluable to
delineate the full extent of the hydrosalpinx and confirm the absence of free
intraperitoneal spill (Fig. 2-16).

Another common diagnostic problem is distinguishing a hydrosalpinx
from a paratubal collection. If there are mucosal folds within a hydrosalpinx
(Fig. 2-17), it is easy to differentiate it from a paratubal collection, which
usually has smooth amorphous walls. Preservation of ampullary mucosal
folds is associated with a better result after tuboplasty. However, as the
ampulla stretches and enlarges, the mucosal folds are effaced (Fig. 2-18).
The dilated ampulla may be composed of several loculated segments, and it
may be impossible to determine where the tubal lumen ends and the

Fig. 2-16. Hysterosal-
pingogram in a 27-year-
old DES daughter with
a history of pelvic infection associated with
an intrauterine device.
A. Huge left hydrosal-
pinx (*H*). Normal right
fallopian tube. B. Drain-
age film and laparotomy
confirmed gigantic left
hydrosalpinx (*H*). (V =
vagina.)

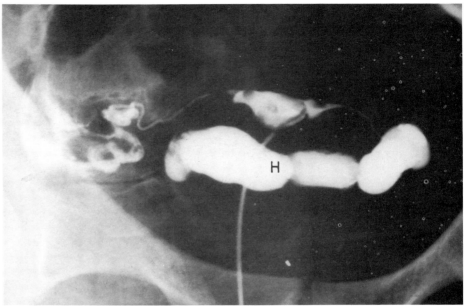

A

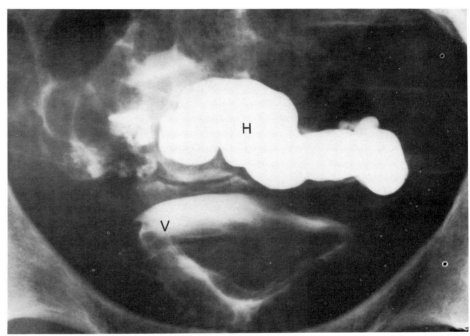

B

Fig. 2-17. Detail of left hydrosalpinx shows prominent mucosal folds (*arrows*) in a patient with past pelvic infection. Surgery showed bilateral obstruction and dilatation of the ampullae. A first-stage tuboplasty was performed.

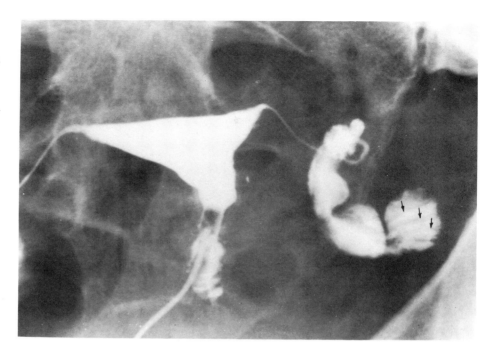

Fig. 2-18. Right cornual obstruction and large left hydrosalpinx (*H*) in a 19-year-old woman with a past history of pelvic inflammatory disease. Overdistension of the ampulla has effaced the mucosal folds and caused intravasation of contrast into the lymphatics (*arrows*) above the hydrosalpinx.

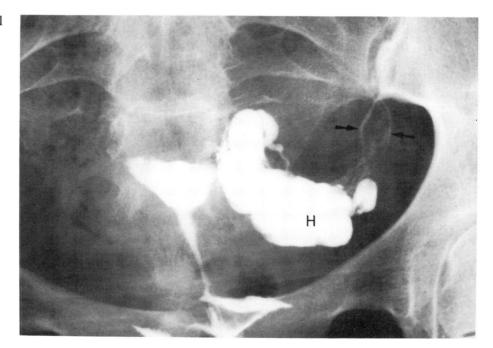

Fig. 2-19. Bilateral hydrosalpinx (*H*) and paratubal collections (*C*). It is impossible to separate the dilated tube from the paratubal cavity. Laparoscopy revealed extensive adhesive endometriosis. (From D. A. Hall and I. C. Yoder, Radiology in the Diagnosis and Therapy of Female Infertility. In J. F. Simeone [ed.], *Coordinated Diagnostic Imaging*. New York: Churchill Livingstone, 1984. Reprinted with permission.)

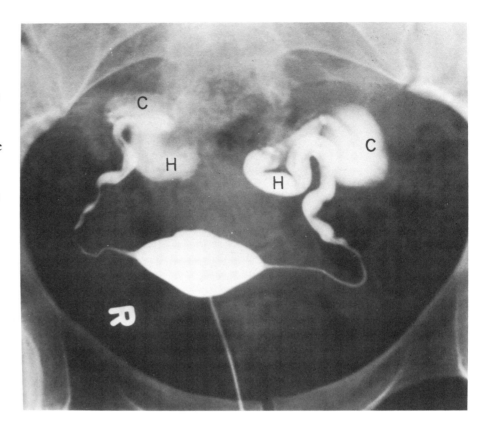

paratubal collection begins (Fig. 2-19). Laparoscopy is the only way to differentiate, which may be of no practical significance since both conditions offer a poor surgical prognosis.

Hydrosalpinx can be unilateral or bilateral. Unilateral tuboovarian abscess has received some attention as a complication of IUD use. Unilateral hydrosalpinx is common, and in a large series only 2 of 36 cases were associated with IUD use [32]. When hydrosalpinx is unilateral, it is extremely important to analyze very precisely the condition of the other tube and ensure its patency and freedom from paratubal adhesions.

Hysterosalpingography may demonstrate an ampullary obstruction without concomitant dilation. These cases probably represent an atrophic form of chronic salpingitis in which the tube is reduced to a thin firm cord with effacement of the mucosal folds and marked atrophy of all of the tubal wall layers [14].

Paratubal Adhesions   Peritoneal adhesions are a common cause of infertility and may develop as a sequela to pelvic inflammatory disease, previous pelvic operations, and endometriosis [28]. Postoperative peritoneal adhesions occur secondary to bleeding, drying of serosal surfaces, use of talc, infection, and tissue necrosis. Patients who have had a previous gynecologic laparotomy performed with conventional operative technique may have a 75 percent rate of adhesions. This indicates the importance of applying very strict criteria for laparotomy in young women and, when necessary, performing laparotomy with atraumatic surgical technique. Adhesions between the tube and the ovary cause sterility by interfering with ovum capture and transport by the fimbria. Even adhesions that appear small and delicate at laparoscopy may cause significant infertility [5].

Hysterosalpingography   Paratubal adhesions and pelvic endometriosis are the lesions most commonly undetected by hysterosalpingography. Some authors have experienced the great frustration of interpreting a hysterosalpingogram as normal with subsequent laparotomy demonstration of paratubal adhesions and have reported a 51.7 percent false-negative rate [8]. Other authors report high accuracy in detecting adhesions on hysterosalpingograms with only a 3 percent false-negative rate [19]. The differences may be caused by technique, authors' experience, and specific disease prevalence in the population. Nevertheless, the latter authors' successes suggest that every effort should be made to diagnose adhesions on hysterosalpingography while remembering the fallibility of the study in this area. Adhesions can be detected on hysterosalpingograms by evidence of delayed or localized contrast spill and abnormal tubal contour. Loculated spill of contrast is seen when contrast spilling out of the fallopian tube remains circumscribed within a boundary adjacent to the tube instead of dispersing freely around bowel loops (Fig. 2-20). Adequate amounts of contrast and drainage films will help demonstrate paratubal collections. Multiple convolutions of the isthmus and ampulla suggest paratubal adhesions, although convolution of the ampulla alone may be normal. It is important to remember that no technique will demonstrate adhesions if these do not interfere with tubal contour or dispersion of contrast from the tube. Similarly adhesions cannot be diagnosed in the presence of tubal occlusion.

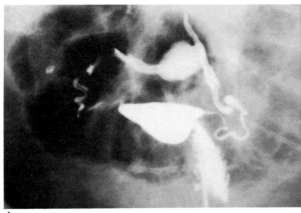

A

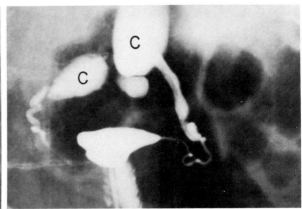

Fig. 2-20. Hysterosal-pingogram in a 32-year-old woman with Crohn's disease, multiple past surgical procedures for adhesions, and 5 years of primary infertility. Bilateral paratubal cavities (*C*) larger on the left side. Following the study the patient developed a temperature of 102° F unresponsive to intravenous antibiotics. Surgery was necessary to drain bilateral *Staphylococcus aureus* abscesses enclosed within extensive pelvic adhesions.

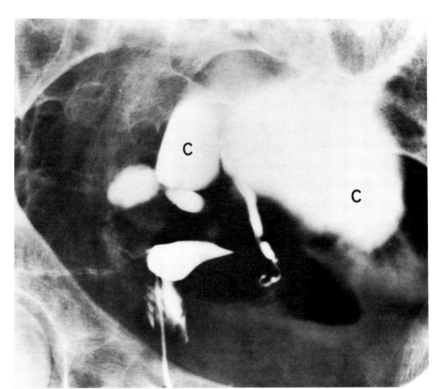

B

Endometriosis

Endometriosis is defined as the presence of benign endometrial epithelium and stroma in an ectopic site. It is estimated that perhaps 15 percent of all women will suffer from endometriosis at some time during their lives. Endometriosis is found at laparoscopy in 6 to 30 percent of infertile female patients [5]. It is more frequent in nulliparous women in their late twenties and thirties and recently has been termed the career woman's disease. The pathogenesis continues to be debated and the major theories are (1) retrograde menstruation and implantation, (2) coelomic metaplasia, and (3) lymphatic or hematogenous dissemination [15]. Endometriosis involves primarily the surfaces of the ovary, uterus, tubes, pelvic ligaments, and cul-de-sac but may occur anywhere in the abdomen. The ectopic implants of endometrium respond to cyclic hormonal fluctuations and undergo proliferation and bleeding. This activity incites inflammation, fibrosis, and adhesions. The symptoms are very variable. Some patients are asymptomatic and diagnosed incidentally at surgery; other patients experience pelvic pain, dysmenorrhea, dyspareunia, and infertility. Symptoms correlate poorly with extent of disease.

Hysterosalpingography

Tubal serosal involvement by endometriosis causes paratubal adhesions, tubal kinking, and altered tubal mobility. The diagnosis of endometriosis can be suggested on hysterosalpingogram when there is evidence of tubal obstruction or adhesions in a patient without a previous history of pelvic infection or surgery (Fig. 2-21). Laparoscopic visualization of pelvic implants provides definitive diagnosis.

Fig. 2-21. Hysterosalpingogram in a 22-year-old woman with pelvic pain and no history of pelvic infection. A. Early film shows a left cornual obstruction and a nondilated but very tortuous ampullary segment of right fallopian tube. B. Later film shows a right paratubal collection (*C*). Laparoscopy demonstrated pelvic endometriosis with extensive adhesions greater on the right side. Indigo carmine dye instillation did not flow through left tube but did flow into right tube and filled a large loculated area of adhesions.

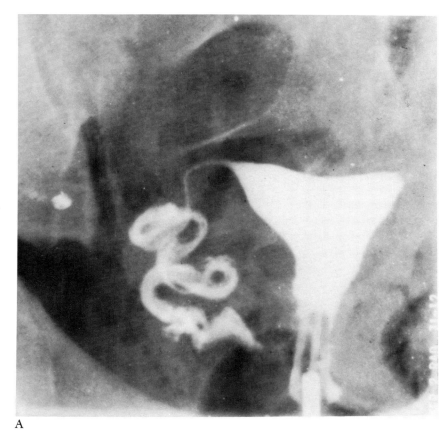

A

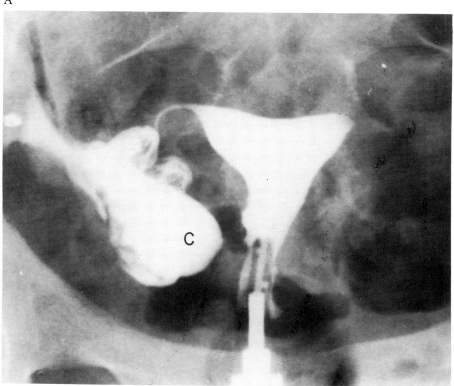

B

Fig. 2-22. Pelvic ultrasound in a 29-year-old woman with a right adnexal mass and a previous left salpingo-oopherectomy for endometriosis. A. Transverse view of the pelvis shows two large masses of variable echogenic texture in the right adnexal region and in the cul-de-sac. B. Sagittal view through the larger of two right adnexal masses. At surgery two large endometriomas were resected along with the uterus and the right fallopian tube. (Courtesy of Dr. Deborah Hall, Boston, Mass.)

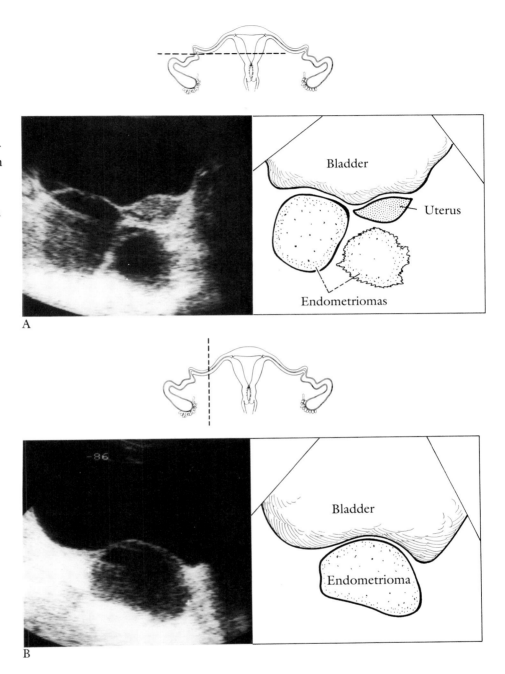

Ultrasound

There are two distinct sonographic patterns of endometriosis: the discrete pelvic mass produced by an endometrioma and the diffuse form associated with multiple focal pelvic implants and adhesions [3]. Endometriomas are characterized by fairly round and discrete adnexal or cul-de-sac masses (Fig. 2-22). These masses may have a cystic, complex, or solid internal pattern. If cystic, a thick wall helps to differentiate them from simple ovarian cysts.

Complex lesions demonstrate low-level echoes or fluid levels representing clots or settling cellular elements within hemorrhagic fluid [13]. Most have a well-defined back wall and enhanced sound transmission characteristic of fluid-filled lesions. Tuboovarian abscesses and hemorrhagic cysts must be included in the differential diagnosis. Solid lesions must be differentiated from neoplasms according to the patient's age and symptoms. In the diffuse form of endometriosis ultrasound may show localized or generalized increase in echogenicity and poor definition of pelvic structures. These are less reliable, nonspecific findings and correlate poorly with the patient's laparoscopic findings [12].

Tubal Tuberculosis   Tuberculosis spreads to the fallopian tubes by hematogenous dissemination from a primary pulmonary focus. Lymphatic spread from mesenteric lymph nodes and direct peritoneal or intestinal extension is also possible. Tuberculosis of the tubes is not considered to be a sexually transmitted infection, although it is theoretically possible for a woman to be infected by a man with tuberculous epididymitis. In the United States tuberculosis accounts for less than 0.01 percent of tubal occlusions found on hysterosalpingography [35]; whereas in a 1972 series from Athens 46 percent of tubal occlusions associated with primary infertility were secondary to tuberculosis [29]. Preliminary plain film of the pelvis may show calcifications of the tubes or ovaries (Fig. 2-23). Genital calcifications are rare and must be differentiated from commonly calcified presacral nodes, calcified uterine myomas, pelvic phleboliths, and the opaque teeth found in ovarian dermoids. Tuberculous tubal abnormalities are almost always bilateral but not symmetric. Caseous ulceration of the mucosa produces ragged contours and diverticular out-pouchings of both the isthmus and the ampulla. Blind-ending sinus tracts and rarely, fistulas to adjacent bowel may form. There may be proliferation of the ampullary mucosal folds, but more often the folds are attenuated, and the ampulla is occluded and either mildly dilated or contracted [40]. Hydrosalpinx is very uncommon. Diverticular cavities may surround the ampulla and give it a characteristic tufted appearance. Isthmic diverticula resemble those seen in salpingitis isthmica nodosa (Fig. 2-24). As tuberculosis heals, the entire tube becomes encased in a heavy connective tissue scar and the lumen develops a beaded, rigid, "pipe stem" appearance. Isthmic obstruction is very frequent and characterized by an irregular patulous lumen (Fig. 2-25). Tubal tuberculosis spreads to the endometrium in approximately one-half of cases, and in these cases the hysterosalpingogram may demonstrate irregularities and scarring of the uterine cavity [34] (Table 2-3). Tuberculous endometrial changes are illustrated in Chapter 4, Diseases of the Uterus.

Fig. 2-23. Tubal tuberculosis. A. Plain film of the pelvis shows calcification of both fallopian tubes (*arrows*). B. Hysterosalpingogram shows interstitial obstruction of both fallopian tubes proximal to calcification. (Courtesy of Drs. H. Tristant and M. Benmussa, Paris, France.)

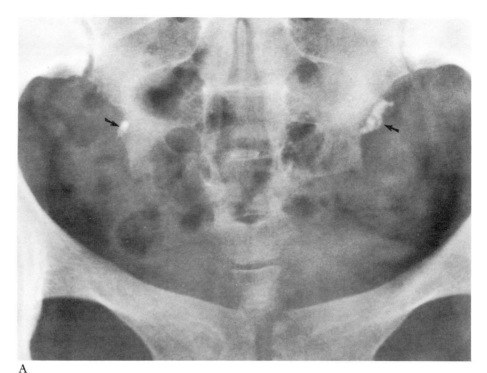

A

B

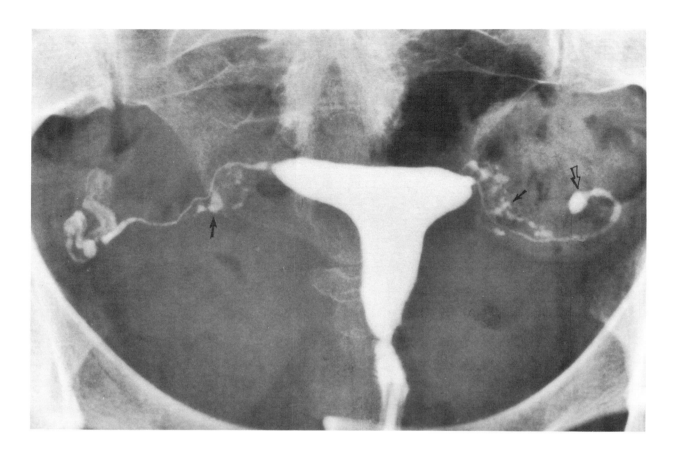

Fig. 2-24. Tubal tuber-
culosis resembling sal-
pingitis isthmica nodosa.
Hysterosalpingogram
demonstrates isthmic di-
verticula (*closed arrows*)
and irregular fallopian
tubes. The left ampulla
is contracted and ob-
structed (*open arrow*).
(Courtesy of Drs. H.
Tristant and M. Ben-
mussa, Paris, France.)

Fig. 2-25. Tubal tuberculosis. Hysterosalpingogram shows rigid, patulous lumina of the isthmic segments of both fallopian tubes. There is isthmic obstruction on the left side and ampullary obstruction on the right side. (Courtesy of Drs. H. Tristant and M. Benmussa, Paris, France.)

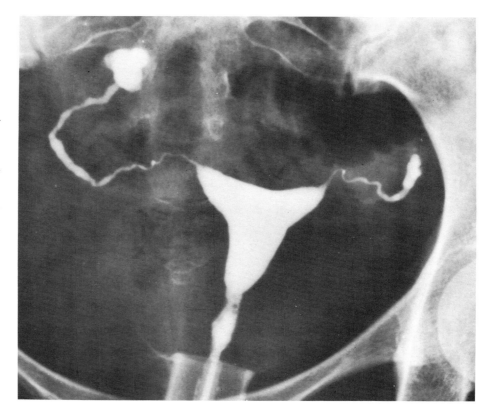

Table 2-3. Characteristics of tubal tuberculosis

Calcification of tubes and ovaries
Occluded and contracted ampulla
Isthmic diverticula and obstruction
Uterine cavity scarring in 50%

Ectopic Pregnancy

Ectopic pregnancy refers to a gestation occurring outside the uterine cavity; 97 percent develop within the fallopian tube [10]. Implantation occurs most often in the ampullary portion, less often in the isthmic portion, and rarely in the interstitial portion of the tube. Other ectopic sites of implantation include the cervix, ovary, and abdominal cavity. The annual incidence of ectopic pregnancy in the United States has increased from 4.8 per 1000 live births (0.5%) in 1970 to 14.1 per 1000 live births (1.5%) in 1980 [20]. Some of this increase is caused by increased numbers of cases of healed salpingitis resulting in tubal deformities that hinder the normal transport of the fertilized ovum. IUDs, therapeutic abortions, endometriosis, and tubal surgery may also promote tubal scarring and increase the risk of ectopic pregnancy. The classic presenting symptoms are pain, abnormal vaginal bleeding, and a pelvic mass. Unfortunately these symptoms are nonspecific, often not present, and easily confused with those of pelvic

Fig. 2-26. Tubal pregnancy. Pelvic ultrasound obtained in a 22-year-old woman with vaginal bleeding and elevated plasma HCG levels. Her last menstrual period occurred 9 weeks before the study. A. Transverse view showed a diffusely enlarged uterus with a decidual reaction, and an ectopic pregnancy within the right tube. Fetus was visible and fetal heart motion was evident. B. Sagittal view through the right tube showed fetus and placenta. At laparoscopy an unruptured right infundibular ectopic pregnancy was removed intact through a salpingostomy. Extensive pelvic adhesions and a clubbed left tube were observed. (Courtesy of Dr. Karen Lindfors, Sacramento, Calif.)

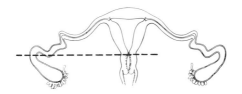

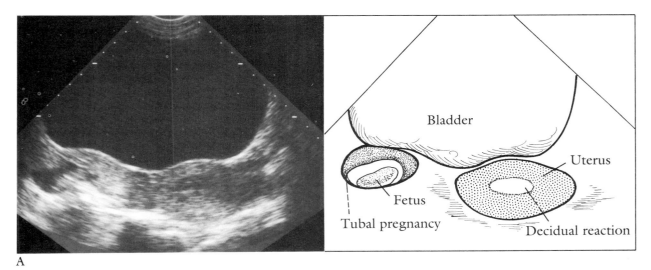

A

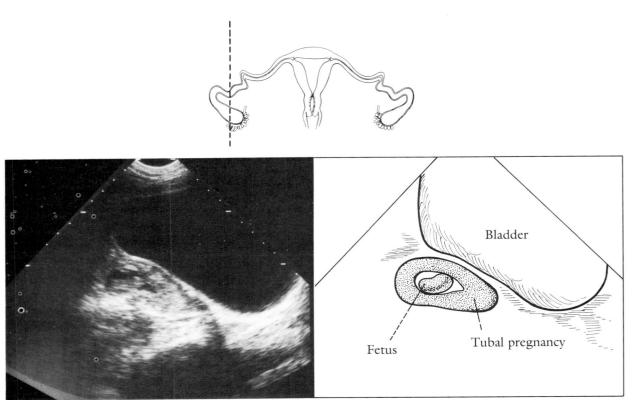

B

inflammatory disease. Tubal rupture is a common and life-threatening event and accounts for 26 percent of all maternal deaths [20].

The diagnosis of tubal pregnancy has always been difficult to establish. Forty years ago hysterosalpingography was sometimes used as a diagnostic aid. In ten cases reported by Marshak in 1946 [24], the ectopic fertilized ovum appeared as a smooth filling defect within a dilated fallopian tube. This report is of interest only because the hysterosalpingogram did not cause rupture of the fallopian tube in any of these patients.

Diagnosis of ectopic pregnancy is now achieved by the combined use of the serum radioimmune assay pregnancy test and high-resolution ultrasonography. Human chorionic gonadotropin (HCG) is produced by placental trophoblastic cells beginning on the eighth day following conception, and under normal circumstances doubles every 2 days until it peaks on the sixth week following conception [1]. Since 1972 a radioimmune assay specific for the beta chain of HCG has enabled accurate qualitative and quantitative detection of small levels of plasma HCG [23]. Simultaneous transabdominal ultrasound examination is routinely obtained in high-risk patients. If the transabdominal sonogram is equivocal, endovaginal ultrasound is recommended. Recent studies suggest that endovaginal sonography can identify intrauterine pregnancies and ectopic gestations earlier than transabdominal sonography [27]. The ultrasound findings in ectopic pregnancy are often difficult to interpret, and early diagnosis requires that the clinician and radiologist maintain a constant high level of suspicion.

The ultrasound is diagnostic of ectopic pregnancy if it demonstrates an extrauterine gestational sac with a viable fetal pole (Fig. 2-26). Unfortunately these unequivocal diagnostic findings are very uncommon. If tubal gestations proceed longer than 6 to 12 weeks, hemorrhage and fetal death are likely. The hemorrhage is secondary to trophoblastic erosion of adjacent blood vessels or tubal rupture. A complex or echogenic adnexal mass can represent a hematosalpinx (Fig. 2-27) composed of a hemorrhagic gestational sac and a dilated blood-filled tube.

Often patients with ectopic pregnancy have nonspecific sonographic findings that include uterine enlargement, an abnormal intrauterine fluid collection, an adnexal mass, and fluid in the cul-de-sac. A cystic adnexal mass is more likely to represent a corpus luteum cyst than an ectopic gestational sac. In one-third of cases the corpus luteum cysts are located on the side opposite that of the ectopic pregnancy [23]. Hemorrhagic ovarian cyst, corpus luteum cyst, pelvic inflammatory disease, and endometriosis can all mimic an ectopic pregnancy. Concurrent fluid in the cul-de-sac increases the probability of ruptured ectopic pregnancy but is also seen in ruptured corpus luteum cyst and tuboovarian abscess.

The demonstration of an intrauterine pregnancy virtually excludes an ectopic pregnancy. Concomitant intrauterine and extrauterine pregnancies are extremely rare; however, their incidence may be increasing from 1 in

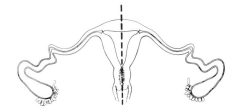

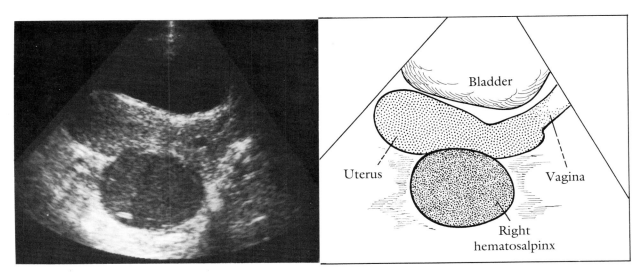

Fig. 2-27. Chronic ectopic pregnancy and hematosalpinx. Pelvic ultrasound obtained in a 27-year-old woman suspected of having an ectopic pregnancy. Sagittal view showed a large, well-circumscribed, echogenic mass behind the uterus. At laparotomy a right tuboovarian mass filled with blood and clots was found posterior to the uterus. Pathologic examination revealed a hematosalpinx with degenerated chorionic villi consistent with an ectopic pregnancy. (Courtesy of Dr. Karen Lindfors, Sacramento, Calif.)

Fig. 2-28. A. Sagittal and (B) transverse pelvic sonograms show an early intrauterine pregnancy. The fetal pole is not visible but a double decidual sac is clearly demonstrated. (Courtesy Dr. Deborah Hall, Boston, Mass.)

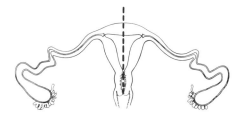

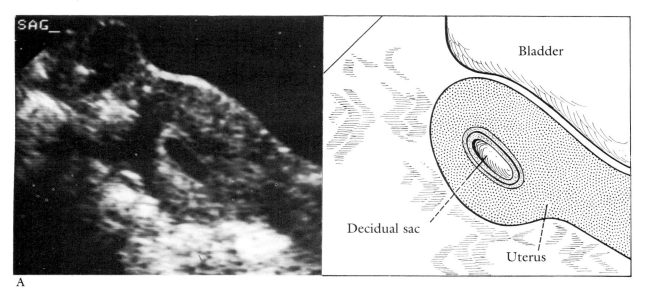

A

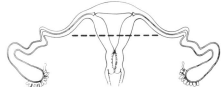

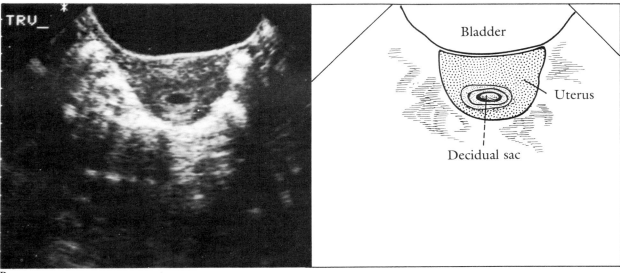

B

Table 2-4. Diagnosis of ectopic pregnancy

Increased levels of plasma HCG
High-resolution abdominal or endovaginal ultrasound
    Extrauterine gestational sac with viable fetal pole
    Decidual cast within uterine cavity (no intrauterine pregnancy)

30,000 to approximately 1 in 7,000 pregnancies (0.014%) along with the general increase in ectopic pregnancy and the use of ovulation-induction agents [18]. An early intrauterine pregnancy shows nonspecific uterine enlargement and decidual thickening on ultrasound until 3 weeks following conception when a gestational sac can be identified, and 5 to 6 weeks following conception when a fetal pole is seen and cardiac activity demonstrated. Prior to visualization of the fetal pole it is difficult to differentiate a true intrauterine gestational sac from a prominent decidual cast, so-called pseudogestational sac, seen in 20 percent of patients with an ectopic pregnancy [1]. Nyberg et al. have described the presence of two concentric rings around a true gestational sac [26]. This double decidual sac is composed of decidua capsularis and decidua parietalis with uterine cavity fluid in between (Fig. 2-28). In contrast, a decidual cast associated with ectopic pregnancy demonstrates fluid surrounded by a single echogenic ring of endometrium undergoing decidual changes. In the Nyberg et al. series 98 percent of patients with a double decidual sac had an intrauterine pregnancy, whereas patients who lacked a double decidual sac were at high risk for an ectopic pregnancy or an abnormal intrauterine pregnancy (blighted ovum or incomplete abortion) [26] (Table 2-4).

There is a linear relation between the sonographic gestational sac size and the exponential rise of serum HCG levels in early pregnancy, before an intrauterine embryo is detected. For example, an HCG level of 6000 mIU/ml* (2nd IS)† corresponds approximately to a gestational sac diameter of 12 mm [25]. This relation falls off at HCG levels above 43,000 mIU/ml (2nd IS) because HCG levels plateau while the sac continues to grow. Failure to find an intrauterine gestational sac at serum HCG levels above 5400 mIU/ml (2nd IS) may suggest ectopic pregnancy or recent spontaneous abortion [10]. However, the discriminatory HCG level will vary according to the resolution of the sonographic equipment and the technique of examination.

---

*Milli-international units per millimeter.
†Second International Standard.

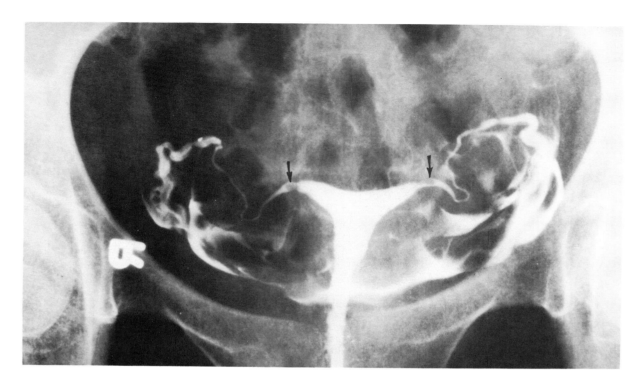

Fig. 2-29. Tubal polyps. Normal hysterosalpingogram shows a small tubal polyp within the interstitial portion of each fallopian tube (*arrows*).

Current efforts at better and earlier detection of ectopic pregnancy are directed toward one goal: prevention of tubal rupture. In addition to reducing maternal morbidity and mortality, early treatment may avoid salpingectomy, allow tubal preservation, and improve future reproductive capability. Microsurgical techniques and conservative tubal surgery, such as linear salpingostomy, have markedly improved subsequent pregnancy rates in patients operated on for unruptured tubal pregnancy [41]. Ectopic pregnancy recurrence is still frequent.

Tubal Polyps

Tubal polyps are small islands of endometrial tissue found within the intramural portion of the fallopian tube. The polyps consist of a benign proliferation of endometrial epithelium and stroma, usually sessile, rarely occurring on a small stalk [14]. They are asymptomatic and present as incidental findings in 1.2 to 2.5 percent of hysterosalpingograms [7]. Tubal polyps appear as smooth bilateral oval filling defects, are less than 1 cm in

Fig. 2-30. Primary adenocarcinoma of the fallopian tube. Hysterosalpingogram shows a dilated left ampulla containing a round tumor mass (*arrows*). (Courtesy of Drs. H. Tristant and M. Benmussa, Paris, France.)

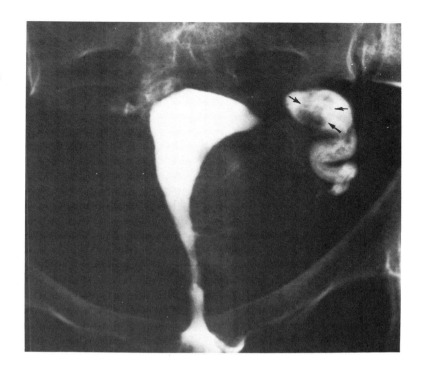

length, and are just beyond the uterine horn (Fig. 2-29). Their presence is subtle and small tubal polyps are easily overlooked since there is no accompanying tubal dilatation or obstruction. A causal relationship between tubal polyps and infertility has been a subject of debate and remains doubtful. The consensus is that other causes of infertility should be searched and treated before microsurgical removal is considered [7].

Tubal Tumors

Tubal cancers are very rare and are more frequently metastatic than primary. Tubal metastases commonly originate from ovarian, endometrial, or cervical carcinomas, infrequently from breast and gastrointestinal sources. Primary adenocarcinoma of the tube arises from the mucosal epithelium and accounts for only 0.5 percent of all malignancies of the female genital tract [14]. Tubal adenocarcinoma is encountered almost exclusively in postmenopausal women (45–65 years), with an occasional occurrence in a younger woman. Hysterosalpingography may demonstrate a bulky, irregular, intraluminal mass within a dilated ampulla (Fig. 2-30). The patient's age will usually differentiate it from an ectopic pregnancy. Localized proliferation of the ampullary mucosa sometimes seen in tuberculous or other chronic salpingitis must be excluded (Fig. 2-31).

Fig. 2-31. Hysterosalpingogram in a 64-year-old woman with a yellow vaginal discharge and left tubal prominence on abdominal computed tomography. The left ampulla has a "cobblestone" mucosal pattern. Contrast spills into a paratubal cavity (C). Surgery revealed sigmoid diverticulitis with a pericolonic abscess and severe adhesions between the left tube and the sigmoid colon. Pathologic examination of the left tube showed acute and chronic salpingitis but no evidence of fistula.

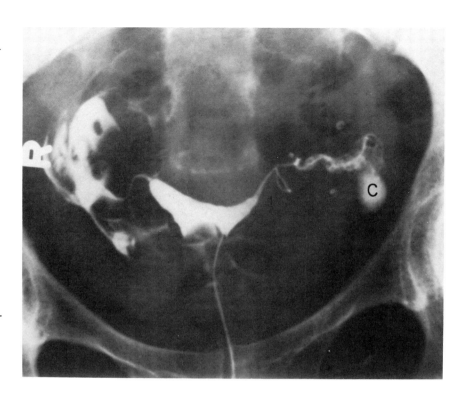

Tubal Fistulas

Fistulas are abnormal passages or communications between a hollow organ and the external surface of the body or between hollow organs. Most fistulas originate from surgical trauma or from an infectious process that disrupts the continuity of the tissues involved. Fallopian tube fistulas most often communicate with the intestine and in more than one-half of the reported cases are secondary to tuberculous salpingitis [33]. Since the incidence of genital tuberculosis is declining, bowel disease and surgery are becoming the more common sources of tubal fistulas. Colonic diverticula, appendicitis, Crohn's disease, and ruptured ectopic pregnancy have produced enterotubal fistulas. Several cases are reported of accidental communication between a peritoneal dialysis cannula and a fallopian tube [4]. A single case of salpingoureteral fistula has been described secondary to ureterolithotomy and subsequent distal ureteral obstruction by recurrent stones [22]. A tubocutaneous (perineum) fistula occurred in a patient following total colectomy for ulcerative colitis [45]. Hysterosalpingography usually demonstrates a dilated, fixed fallopian tube and spill of contrast into an abnormal site. Delayed films help to confirm flow into intestine, perineum, or ureter. Intestinal barium study or contrast infusion into a sinus tract or peritoneal cannula often demonstrates the abnormal communication and outlines the fallopian tubes and uterus.

Other Studies

Radionuclide and ultrasound studies have been used on a small scale to evaluate tubal function and to assess the patency of the fallopian tubes. Human albumin microspheres labeled with technetium 99m and suspended in 1 ml of saline were deposited in the vaginal fornix and external os of female volunteers and imaged serially with a gamma camera [36]. Within 15 to 30 minutes radioactivity was observed in the uterus and tubes and spreading over the ovaries. This study confirms the prompt spontaneous migration of inert particles from the vagina to the peritoneum and as such may serve as an index of tubal function. The resolution of the images obtained is inferior to hysterosalpingography images, but the technique may be useful in the postoperative evaluation of tubal function in the future.

Sonosalpingography is the introduction of sterile fluid into the uterus followed by ultrasound evaluation of the pelvis to document fluid in the cul-de-sac, indicating at least unilateral tubal patency [31]. This study avoids exposure to ionizing radiation but cannot define tubal anatomic structure.

References

1. Athey, P. A. Ectopic Pregnancy. In P. A. Athey and F. P. Hadlock (eds.), *Ultrasound in Obstetrics and Gynecology* (2nd ed.). St. Louis: Mosby, 1985. Pp. 251–271.
2. Athey, P. A. Pelvic Inflammatory Disease. In P. A. Athey and F. P. Hadlock (eds.), *Ultrasound in Obstetrics and Gynecology* (2nd ed.). St. Louis, Mosby, 1985. Pp. 239–250.
3. Birnholz, J. C. Endometriosis and inflammatory disease. *Semin. Ultrasound* 4:184, 1983.
4. Chatterton, B. Communication between a continuous ambulatory peritoneal dialysis cannula and right fallopian tube demonstrated radiographically. *Br. J. Radiol.* 57:924, 1984.
5. Corson, S. L. Uses of the laparoscope in the infertile patient comparative study. *Fertil. Steril.* 32:359, 1979.
6. Creasy, J. L., et al. Salpingitis isthmica nodosa: radiologic and clinical correlates. *Radiology* 154:597, 1985.
7. David, M. P., Ben-Zwi, D., and Langer, L. Tubal intramural polyps and their relationship to infertility. *Fertil. Steril.* 35:526, 1981.
8. Duff, D. E., et al. Hysterosalpingography and laparoscopy: a comparative study. *AJR* 141:761, 1983.
9. Eschenbach, D. A., Harnisch, J. P., and Holmes, K. K. Pathogenesis of acute pelvic inflammatory disease: role of contraception and other risk factors. *Am. J. Obstet. Gynecol.* 128:838, 1977.
10. Filly, R. A. Ectopic pregnancy: the role of sonography. *Radiology* 162:661, 1987.
11. Fortier, K. J., and Haney, A. F. A pathologic spectrum of uretero-tubal junction obstruction. *Obstet. Gynecol.* 65:93, 1985.

12. Friedman, H., et al. Endometriosis detection by US with laparoscopic correlation. *Radiology* 157:217, 1985.
13. Goldman, S. M., and Minkin, S. I. Diagnosing endometriosis with ultrasound. Accuracy and specificity. *J. Reprod. Med.* 25:178, 1980.
14. Gompel, C., and Silverberg, S. G. *Pathology in Gynecology and Obstetrics* (3rd ed.). Philadelphia: Lippincott, 1985. Pp. 278–305.
15. Gompel, C., and Silverberg, S. G. *Pathology in Gynecology and Obstetrics* (3rd ed.). Philadelphia: Lippincott, 1985. Pp. 403–434.
16. Halbert, S. A. Function and Structure of the Fallopian Tube. In V. Gomel (ed.), *Microsurgery in Female Infertility*. Boston: Little, Brown, 1983. Pp. 7–27.
17. Hall, D. A., and Yoder, I. C. Radiology in the Diagnosis and Therapy of Female Infertility. In J. F. Simeone (ed.), *Coordinated Diagnostic Imaging*. New York: Churchill Livingstone, 1984. Pp. 111–140.
18. Hann, L. E., Bachman, D. M., and McArdle, C. R. Coexistent intrauterine and ectopic pregnancy: a re-evaluation. *Radiology* 152:151, 1984.
19. Horwitz, R. C., Morton, P. C. G., and Shaff, M. I. A radiological approach to infertility—hysterosalpingography. *Br. J. Radiol.* 52:255, 1979.
20. James, E. A., et al. Ectopic pregnancy: a malpractice paradigm. *Radiology* 160:411, 1986.
21. Karasick, S., Karasick, D., and Schilling, J. Salpingitis isthmica nodosa in female infertility. *J. Can. Assoc. Radiol.* 36:118, 1985.
22. Keegan, G. T., and Turner, W. R. A case report: salpingoureteral fistula. *J. Urol.* 115:218, 1976.
23. Laing, F. C., and Jeffrey, R. B. Ultrasound evaluation of ectopic pregnancy. *Radiol. Clin. North Am.* 20:383, 1982.
24. Marshak, R. Radiologic diagnosis of ectopic pregnancy. *N.Y. State J. Med.* 46:317, 1946.
25. Nyberg, D. A., et al. Early gestation: correlation of HCG levels and sonographic identification. *AJR* 144:951, 1985.
26. Nyberg, D. A., et al. Ultrasonographic differentiation of the gestational sac of early intrauterine pregnancy from the pseudogestational sac of ectopic pregnancy. *Radiology* 146:755, 1983.
27. Nyberg, D. A., et al. Endovaginal sonographic evaluation of ectopic pregnancy: A prospective study. *AJR* 149:1181, 1987.
28. Patton, G. W., and Kistner, R. W. Surgery of the Oviduct. In *Atlas of Infertility Surgery* (2nd ed.). Boston: Little, Brown, 1984. Pp. 213–310.
29. Pontifex, G., Trichopoulos, D., and Karpathios, S. Hysterosalpingography in the diagnosis of infertility. *Fertil. Steril.* 23:829, 1972.
30. Punnonen, R., and Soderstrom, K. O. Inflammatory etiology of salpingitis isthmica nodosa: a clinical, histological and ultrastructural study. *Acta Eur. Fertil.* 17:199, 1986.
31. Richman, T. S., et al. Fallopian tubal patency assessed by ultrasound following fluid injection. *Radiology* 152:507, 1984.
32. San Filippo, J. S., Yussman, M. A., and Smith, O. Hysterosalpingography in the evaluation of infertility: 6 year review. *Fertil. Steril.* 30:636, 1978.

33. Sbihi, H., Muntlak, H., and Tubiana, J. M. Tubo-intestinal fistulae. *Ann. Radiol. (Paris)* 23:565, 1980.
34. Siegler, A. M. *Hysterosalpingography* (2nd ed.). New York: Medcom, 1974. Pp. 125–139.
35. Siegler, A. M., and Kontopoulos, V. Female genital tuberculosis and the role of hysterosalpingography. *Semin. Radiol.* 14:295, 1979.
36. Stone, S. C., et al. Radionuclide evaluation of tubal function. *Fertil. Steril.* 43:757, 1985.
37. Swayne, L. C., Love, M. B., and Karasick, S. R. Pelvic inflammatory disease: sonographic-pathologic correlation. *Radiology* 151:751, 1984.
38. Sweet, R. L., et al. The occurrence of chlamydial and gonococcal salpingitis during the menstrual cycle. *J.A.M.A.* 255:2062, 1986.
39. Thurmond, A. S., et al. Fallopian tube obstruction: selective salpingography and recanalization. *Radiology* 163:511, 1987.
40. Tristant, H., and Benmussa, M. *Atlas d'Hysterosalpingographie.* Paris: Masson, 1981. Pp. 239–258.
41. Weckstein, L. N., et al. Accurate diagnosis of early ectopic pregnancy. *Obstet. Gynecol.* 65:393, 1985.
42. Westrom, L. Effect of acute pelvic inflammatory disease on fertility. *Am. J. Obstet. Gynecol.* 121:707, 1975.
43. Westrom L. Incidence, prevalence, and trends of acute pelvic inflammatory disease and its consequences in industrialized countries. *Am. J. Obstet. Gynecol.* 138:880, 1980.
44. Westrom, L. Influence of sexually transmitted disease on sterility and ectopic pregnancy. *Acta Eur. Fertil.* 16:21, 1985.
45. Wittick, A. C., Morales, H., and Braeuer, N. R. Tubocutaneous fistula. *Am. J. Obstet. Gynecol.* 144:109, 1982.
46. World Health Organization. A new hysterographic approach of tubal spasm and spasmolytic agents. *Fertil. Steril.* 39:105, 1983.

Fig. 3-3. Pomeroy tubal ligation. Hysterosalpingogram performed prior to tubal reconstruction shows relatively long and slender isthmic segments of both tubes. There is an abrupt surgical occlusion near the isthmoampullary junction on both sides (*arrows*).

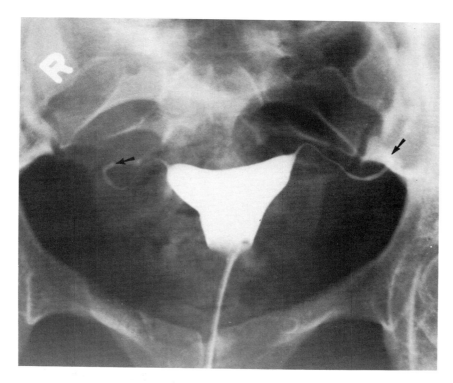

Hysterosalpingography. The hysterosalpingogram has been used extensively in the postoperative evaluation of new methods of surgical tubal sterilization [3,13,23]. Once the efficacy of a new method of sterilization is established, the study is used only to confirm tubal occlusion in surgically difficult cases in which the success of the occlusion is in doubt. Presently the primary reason for a postligation hysterosalpingogram is surgical reversal. Prior to tubal reanastomosis the hysterosalpingogram is used to delineate the length and condition of the proximal tubal segment.

When used to evaluate the success of tubal occlusion, the hysterosalpingogram should be performed 12 weeks or more after surgery to ensure that the operative site is fully fibrosed and that contrast instilled into the uterus at moderate pressures will not produce a tuboperitoneal fistula. Following tubal ligation by the Pomeroy or Irving techniques, electrocoagulation, or mechanical devices, the majority of blocked tubes show an abrupt end to the passage of contrast several centimeters lateral to the uterine horn. The tubal lumen is either normal in caliber (Fig. 3-3) or has a bulbous dilatation proximal to the site of isthmic occlusion (Fig. 3-4). The hysterosalpingogram may also demonstate cornual obstruction in patients who have had an isthmic ligation (Fig. 3-5). Failure to fill the isthmic segment may be secondary to reactive luminal fibrosis or caused by blockage of the lumen by tubal secretions [3].

Infrequently contrast extravasates from the tube into a small localized area of adhesions at the site of ligation (Fig. 3-6). This appearance is con-

Fig. 3-4. Falope ring tubal ligation. Preoperative hysterosalpingogram shows short and slightly dilated isthmic segment. Each tube measures approximately 4 cm from the interstitial mucosal fold to the site of occlusion. This length is ample to accomplish a successful tubal reanastomosis.

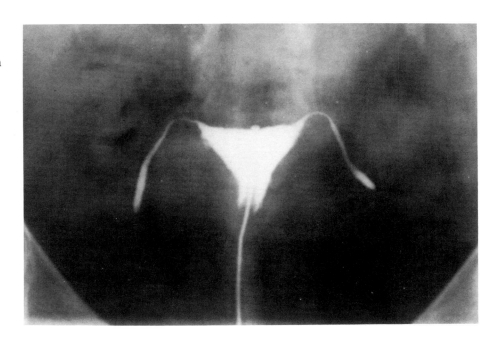

Fig. 3-5. Hysterosalpingogram in a 34-year-old woman 5 years after tubal ligation. Falope rings seen en face (*arrows*). The left tube filled to the level of the midisthmic ligation. The right tube did not fill beyond the interstitial segment.

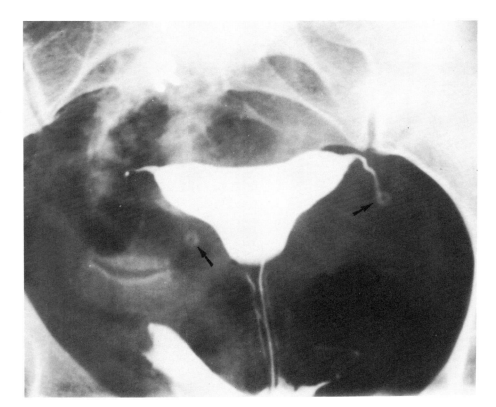

Fig. 3-6. Hysterosalpingogram 2 months after Falope ring tubal ligations rendered difficult by the presence of heavy adhesions. The study shows bilateral midisthmic tubal occlusion and a localized extravasation of contrast at the left surgical site (*arrow*).

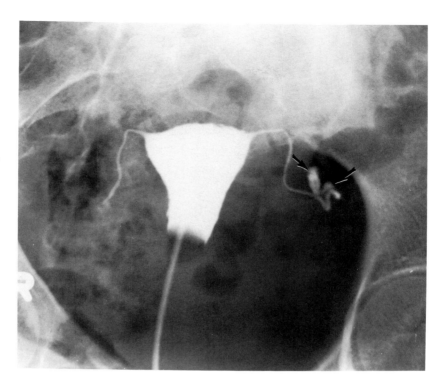

sistent with a successful occlusion. However, if there is free intraperitoneal spill at the site of ligation, a tuboperitoneal fistula is present (Fig. 3-7). In this situation a patient can become pregnant and alternative contraception is advised until a repeat study 4 to 6 weeks later documents closure of the fistula [23]. If the fistula persists on the second study a repeat sterilization is usually performed. Intravasation of contrast into venous and lymphatic channels is quite common in the presence of bilateral tubal occlusion and should not be misinterpreted as free peritoneal dispersion (Fig. 3-8).

Following fimbriectomy, contrast fills the fallopian tube beyond the isthmus into a dilated, shortened, and completely obstructed ampulla (Fig. 3-9). Following the Irving procedure, the isthmic portion of the tube may show a sharp downward angulation instead of the straight course seen after the other occlusive procedures [26].

Very rarely a normal appearing tube with free intraperitoneal spill is detected after a tubal ligation. This appearance suggests that the round ligament was mistakenly ligated instead of the fallopian tube, that the ligature has fallen off, or less likely, that tubal recanalization has occurred after successful ligation.

Hulka clips have metallic hinges and are easily seen on plain radiographs of the pelvis. Falope rings are more difficult to identify on plain films [17,24]. The silastic rings are seen within the true pelvis (Fig. 3-10) as two perfectly rounded radiopaque densities with central lucencies. They are less

Fig. 3-7. Hysterosalpingogram after recent Pomeroy tubal ligation shows bilateral isthmic occlusions (*arrows*). There is free peritoneal spill of contrast on the left side. The tuboperitoneal fistula originates in the mid-isthmus at the site of surgical occlusion. (From D. A. Hall and I. C. Yoder, Radiology in the Diagnosis and Therapy of Female Infertility. In J. F. Simeone [ed.], *Coordinated Diagnostic Imaging*. New York: Churchill Livingstone, 1984. Reprinted with permission.)

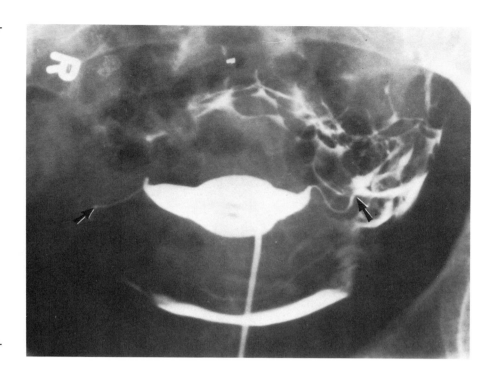

Fig. 3-8. Hysterosalpingogram shows bilateral isthmic occlusion to falope ring (*white arrows*). Extensive venous intravasation occurred on both sides (*black arrows*). Veins should not be confused with distal tubes or free intraperitoneal spill.

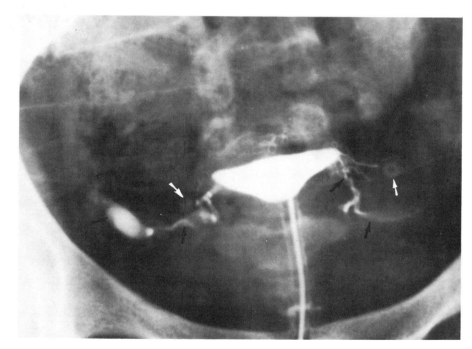

Fig. 3-9. Hysterosalpingogram several years after fimbriectomy shows bilateral ampullary obstruction and no free intraperitoneal spill. Note venous intravasation on left side (*arrows*).

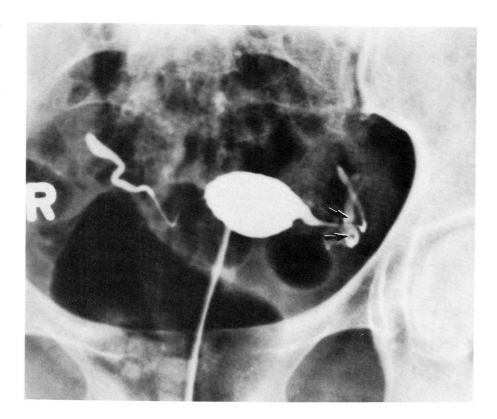

Fig. 3-10. Plain film of the pelvis shows the opaque falope rings. The right ring is seen end-on and has a central lucency (*open arrow*). The left ring is seen on its side and the central lucency is not visible (*closed arrow*).

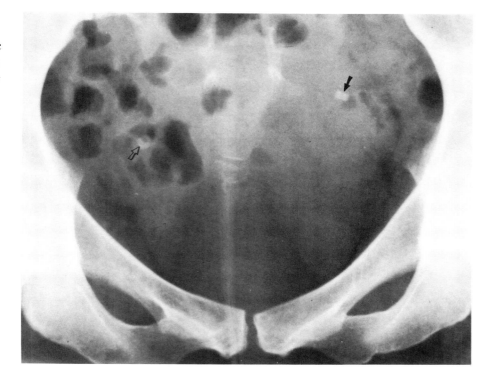

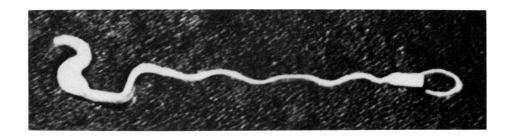

Fig. 3-11. Removed silicone plug. (From S. J. Dan and M. S. Goldstein. Fallopian tube occlusion with silicone: radiographic appearance. *Radiology* 151:603, 1984. Reprinted with permission.)

dense but can be mistaken for pelvic phleboliths or ureteral calculi. Pelvic phleboliths also have central lucencies but are not as medially located or as smooth as silastic rings. Ureteral calculi are unlikely to be bilateral and symmetric or to have central lucencies.

Hysteroscopic Sterilization

Hysteroscopic sterilization is in its infancy but is likely to gain favor within the next decade. Techniques for hysteroscopic sterilization can be divided into two main groups: (1) destructive techniques in which the tubal ostia are destroyed by electrocoagulation or the use of chemical sclerosing substances such as quinacrine or methylcyanoacrylate [8]; and (2) nondestructive techniques in which the tubes are occluded by introducing a plug or other substance through the tubal ostia. Methylcyanoacrylate produces irreversible fibrotic changes within the tubes. It is presently being extensively tested as a method of female sterilization in Brazil, Chile, and Venezuela. Formed-in-place silicone rubber plugs are a promising nondestructive technique developed by Erb in 1978 presently undergoing widespread clinical trials in the United States [21].

Silicone Occlusion of Fallopian Tubes

Under hysteroscopic control a silicone rubber obturator tip is placed in the tubal ostium and used to pump liquid silicone polymer and a catalyst into the oviduct [21]. The mixture contains spherical silver powder, which renders it radiopaque. The material solidifies in situ and conforms to the shape of the tubal lumen. The obturator tip is bonded to the formed-in-place silicone plug and has a metal loop that allows subsequent hysteroscopic removal (Fig. 3-11).

To date successful bilateral tubal plug placement has been feasible in up to 86 percent of patients, and future instrument improvements should increase these rates [14]. The procedure can be performed on an outpatient basis under paracervical block regional anesthesia. Immediately after the procedure the patient has a plain film radiograph of the pelvis to confirm adequate formation of the tubal plugs.

Fig. 3-12. Angled view of the pelvis shows correctly formed silicone plugs. (Courtesy of Dr. Sol J. Dan, New York, N.Y.)

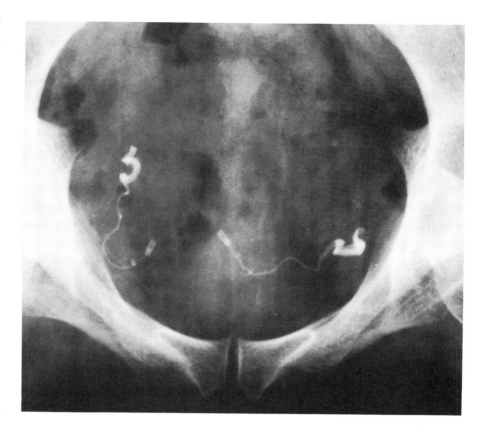

Radiography. On x ray the normal silicone plug provides a radiopaque cast of the tubal lumen with an enlarged ampullary portion, a thin isthmus, and a thick obturator tip [4,6]. The entire plug should be continuous, and oblique films may be necessary to demonstrate continuity in very tortuous fallopian tubes (Fig. 3-12). Abnormally formed plugs can (1) be discontinuous, (2) have a typical extravasated appearance, (3) lack the normal widening at the ampulla (Fig. 3-13), and (4) show displacement of the distal segment into the peritoneal cavity [4]. A plug remains in place because of the anchoring provided at each end by the ampullary widening and the obturator tip. If there is a break in continuity the plug segments will fall into the uterine and peritoneal cavities. Injection of the silicone solution into the myometrium or uterine veins will result in abnormal accumulation of radiopaque material in the uterine wall [6] (Fig. 3-14). This extravasated appearance alerts the physician that the plug cannot be relied on for contraception. Absence of normal expansion of the ampullary portion of the plug is probably caused by intrinsic tubal abnormality and makes retention unlikely.

Fig. 3-13. Plain film of the pelvis shows lack of ampullary widening of the left silicone plug (*arrow*). Normally formed right plug. (From S. J. Dan and M. S. Goldstein. Fallopian tube occlusion with silicone: radiographic appearance. *Radiology* 151:603, 1984. Reprinted with permission.)

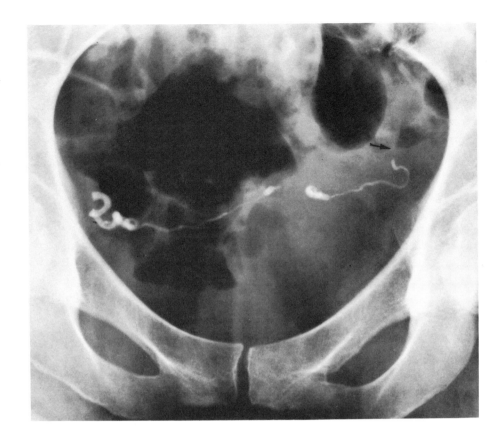

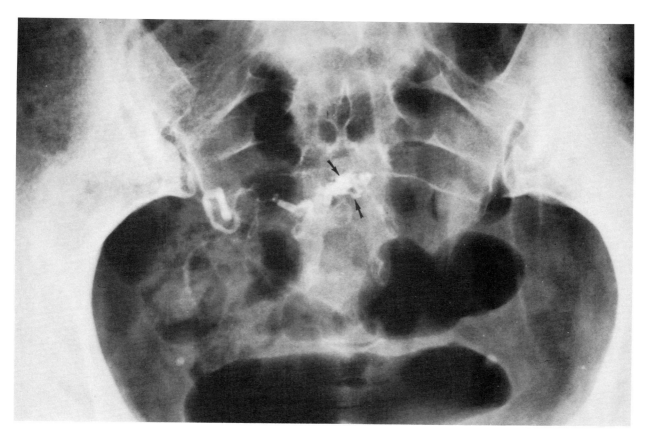

Fig. 3-14. Plain film of the pelvis shows extravasation of silicone into the proximal left peritubal space (*arrows*). Normally formed right plug. (From S. J. Dan and M. S. Goldstein. Fallopian tube occlusion with silicone: radiographic appearance. *Radiology* 151:603, 1984. Reprinted with permission.)

Fig. 3-15. Plain film of the abdomen shows a peritoneal first plug (*arrow*) adjacent to a normally formed second right silicone plug. The left plug is normal. (From S. J. Dan and M. S. Goldstein. Fallopian tube occlusion with silicone: radiographic appearance. *Radiology* 151:603, 1984. Reprinted with permission.)

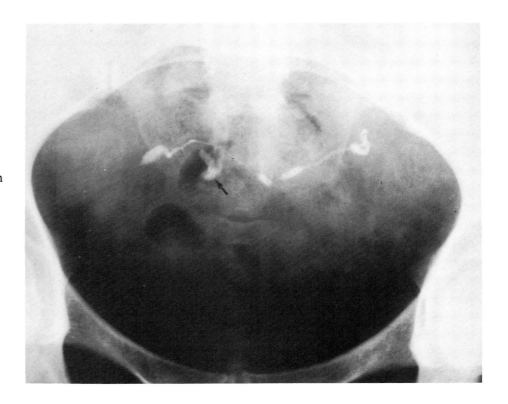

Additional radiographs are obtained 3 months and 2 years after silicone plug placement to confirm continued normal appearance. These films may demonstrate migration of the tubal portion of the plug into the peritoneal cavity. Migration is caused by either an accidental separation of the plug or intentional plug removal by a physician. Plug removal is accomplished by hysteroscopic separation of the obturator tip from the rest of the plug. Only the obturator tip can be retrieved and the remainder of the plug falls into the peritoneal cavity (Fig. 3-15).

The radiographic appearance of silicone tubal plugs is fairly characteristic and should be easily differentiated from pelvic calcifications and contrast from a recent hysterosalpingogram. Since the silicone plugs are radiopaque, hysterosalpingogram is never indicated after successful insertion. The study may be needed preoperatively when tubal abnormality, which might interfere with plug placement, is suspected, or after misplacement if a second plug introduction is going to be attempted [21].

The tubal occlusion provided by silicone plugs is potentially reversible since silicone is an inert material that does not harm the endosalpinx. Although small clinical trials have shown reversibility in animals, proof of reversibility in human beings awaits more widespread use of the method.

Tubal Reconstruction	Microsurgical techniques are standard practice for all gynecologic infertility procedures today [10,20,27]. Although the operating microscope has been available for over 40 years, its use in pelvic surgery has flourished only during the past decade. High magnification enables the surgeon to differentiate normal tissue from abnormal tissue and allows precise anastomosis of the fallopian tube, especially the extremely narrow caliber intramural segment. Microsurgery utilizes the gentle handling of tissues and uses fine inert suture material, specialized atraumatic instruments, warmed isotonic solutions for continuous irrigation, and meticulous hemostasis [10]. The purpose is to minimize direct injury to the fallopian tube and to prevent the development of postoperative adhesions. The microsurgical approach has resulted in an increased success rate of tuboplasty; overall term pregnancy rates have doubled compared with that of conventional tubal surgery, and the ectopic pregnancy rates have decreased considerably [20]. The results of microsurgical reconstruction of the fallopian tubes vary according to the underlying tubal pathology. A pregnancy rate of up to 95 percent can be attained in reversal of clip or ring tubal sterilization [18] where tissue damage was localized to a small section of isthmus. In contrast a 34 percent pregnancy rate is the best result reported in patients with diffuse tubal inflammatory changes who are undergoing repair of bilateral chronic hydrosalpinx [19]. Thus microsurgery can restore tubal patency, but other coexisting pathologic changes within and around the fallopian tube may interfere with its function and prevent subsequent conception and/or successful pregnancy.

Surgical Techniques

The International Society of Fertility has classified surgical procedures of the fallopian tube into lysis of adhesions, fimbrioplasty, salpingoneostomy, tubotubal anastomosis, uterotubal anastomosis, linear salpingotomy, and combinations [20] (Table 3-1). Salpingolysis and ovariolysis, the removal of adhesions surrounding the fallopian tube and ovary, are sometimes performed alone but more often accompany almost all tubal repair procedures. Fimbrioplasty is the separation of adherent fimbria in a nonoccluded tube; salpingoneostomy (salpingostomy) is the repair of a dilated and totally occluded distal tube. Tubotubal anastomoses can be performed at any level and are in increasing demand for reversal of tubal ligations. Tubouterine implantations have been discontinued with the advent of microsurgical techniques that allow uterotubal anastomoses [20,27].

Linear salpingotomy is a horizontal incision over the dilated portion of the fallopian tube containing an unruptured ectopic pregnancy [12]. The products of conception are evacuated, bleeding is controlled, and the incision is either sutured closed or left open and allowed to heal by primary intention [5]. Linear salpingotomy is rapidly becoming an accepted way to manage early tubal pregnancy because it allows removal of the products of conception without destruction of the tube [12].

Table 3-1. Classification of tubal surgery

Lysis of adhesions
   Salpingolysis and/or ovariolysis
Fimbrioplasty
Salpingoneostomy (salpingostomy)
Tubotubal anastomosis
Uterotubal anastomosis
Linear salpingotomy
Combinations

Hysterosalpingography

Postoperative hysterosalpingography is used primarily for patients who remain infertile following tubal reconstruction. The study confirms restoration of tubal patency and evaluates the other factors that interfere with postoperative fertility. These factors include destruction of the tubal mucosa, marked shortening of the oviduct, and persistent or new pelvic adhesions [9].

Fimbrioplasty and Salpingoneostomy

The repair of a hydrosalpinx continues to produce few successful pregnancies. After fimbrioplasty or salpingoneostomy, more than one-half of the hysterosalpingograms reveal persistent dilatation and occlusion of the ampulla [22] (Fig. 3-16). Reocclusion may be secondary to poor surgical technique, but it is more likely primarily related to the severity of the underlying pathology. However, even patients who have patent tubes often fail to conceive [9]. This failure is very likely caused by destruction of the ciliated cells of tubal mucosa by previous infection. The normal tubal mucosa consists of a single layer of columnar epithelium primarily composed of ciliated and secretory cells [7]. The ciliated cells are more numerous in the fimbria and ampulla and progressively decrease in number toward the isthmus. Estrogen causes the cilia to beat actively toward the uterus and carry the egg cumulus into the ostium and through the ampulla. Permanent destruction of ciliated cells will interfere with ovum pick-up and transport. Electron microscopy study of tubal biopsies shows that as the number of ciliated cells decreases, the frequency of uterine pregnancies also decreases and the number of ectopic pregnancies increases [25].

Although the hysterosalpingogram is unable to demonstrate microscopic changes in the tubal epithelium, it can accurately depict the presence or absence of normal ampullary mucosal folds. Patients with normal appearing mucosal folds on hysterosalpingography have a much higher rate of pregnancy (65%) than patients without mucosal folds (7%) [20]. A normal postoperative mucosal pattern is also likely to have a direct correlation with the rate of subsequent intrauterine pregnancy.

Fig. 3-20. Hysterosalpingograms pre- and post-right salpingoneostomy and left uterotubal implantation. A. Preoperative study showed right hydrosalpinx (*H*) and left interstitial obstruction. B. One year after surgery the right ampulla was markedly decreased in size but adhesions caused contrast to accumulate in a paratubal collection (*C*). Left interstitial obstruction persists.

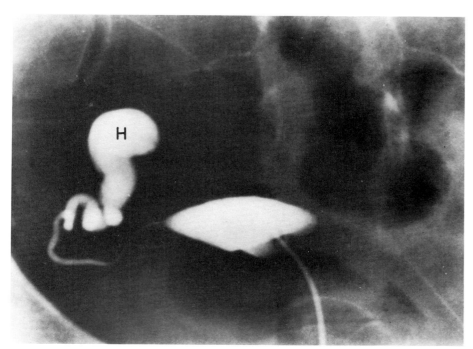

A

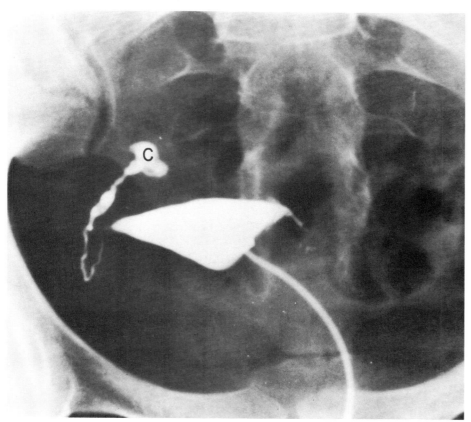

B

| Uterotubal Anastomosis | After successful uterotubal anastomosis, the hysterosalpingogram shows widening of the luminal diameter of the site of anastomosis and variable shortening of the tube [22]. |

| Linear Salpingotomy | Following linear salpingotomy, the hysterosalpingogram may show peritoneal extravasation of contrast at the site of surgery with blunting and obstruction of the distal ampulla (Fig. 3-19). Alternatively the surgical site closes, and there is variable ampullary dilatation with or without peritoneal spill. |

| Adhesions | Paratubal adhesions are common in postoperative hysterosalpingograms. Extensive dense adhesions tend to reform following surgical lysis and new adhesions may occur despite meticulous surgical techniques (Fig. 3-20). Periadnexal adhesions may encase the ovary and fimbria together or may result in extreme spatial separation between the tube and ovary. In either case adhesions interfere with the ability of the tube to capture the egg cumulus as it is extruded from the surface of the ovary into the peritoneal cavity. |

References

1. Ansari, A. M., Marik, J. J., and Moore, J. G. Laparoscopic Tubal Sterilization. In A. M. Siegler (ed.), *The Fallopian Tube*. Mount Kisco: Futura Publishing Co., Inc., 1986. Pp. 307–309.
2. Barwin, B. N. Tubal Sterilization at Laparotomy. In A. M. Siegler (ed.), *The Fallopian Tube*. Mount Kisco: Futura Publishing Co., Inc., 1986. Pp. 321–328.
3. Beck, P., Gal, D., and Tancer, M. L. Silicone band sterilization with radiographic and laparoscopic evaluation. *Obstet. Gynecol.* 53:698, 1979.
4. Dan, S. J., and Goldstein, M. S. Fallopian tube occlusion with silicone: radiographic appearance. *Radiology* 151:603, 1984.
5. DeCherney, A. H., Maheaux, R., and Naftolin, F. Salpingostomy for ectopic pregnancy in the sole patent oviduct: reproductive outcome. *Fertil. Steril.* 37:619, 1982.
6. Fischer, M. E., Reed, T. P., and Red, D. E. Silicone devices for tubal occlusion: Radiographic description and evaluation. *Radiology* 151:601, 1984.
7. Fredericks, C. M. Morphological and Functional Aspects of the Oviductal Epithelium. In A. M. Siegler (ed.), *The Fallopian Tube*. Mount Kisco: Futura Publishing Co., Inc., 1986. Pp. 67–80.
8. Goldsmith, A. The use of methylcyanoacrylate (MCA) for female sterilization. *Contraception* 31:243, 1985.
9. Gomel, V. Causes of failed tubal microsurgery. *J. Reprod. Med.* 24:239, 1980.
10. Gomel, V. *Microsurgery in Female Infertility*. Boston: Little, Brown, 1983. Pp. 147–149.
11. Gomel, V. *Microsurgery in Female Infertility*. Boston: Little, Brown, 1983. Pp. 225–251.

12. Gomel, V. *Microsurgery in Female Infertility.* Boston: Little, Brown, 1983. Pp. 253–265.

13. Hertz, J. B. Laparoscopic sterilization with the falope-ring technique. *Acta Obstet. Gynecol. Scand.* 61:13, 1982.

14. Houck, R. M., and Cooper, J. M. Hysteroscopic tubal occlusion with formed-in-place silicone plugs. *Obstet. Gynecol.* 60:641, 1982.

15. Higgins, G. R., and Sondheimer, S. J. Complications of female sterilization: Immediate and delayed. In E. E. Wallach and R. D. Kempus (eds.), *Modern Trends in Infertility and Conception Control.* Chicago: Year Book, Inc., 1985. Pp. 492–509.

16. Hulka, J. F., et al. Laparoscopic sterilization with the spring clip: Instrumentation development and current clinical experience. *Am. J. Obstet. Gynecol.* 135:1016, 1979.

17. McJunkin, M. L., and Curtis, J. A. Radiographic appearance of laparoscopic tubal ring. *AJR* 132:297, 1979.

18. Owen, E. Reversal of female sterilization. Review of 252 microsurgical salpingo-salpingostomies. *Med. J. Aust.* 141:276, 1984.

19. Owen, E., and Ansari, A. H. Tubal Microsurgery. In A. M. Siegler (ed.), *The Fallopian Tube.* Mount Kisco: Futura Publishing Co., Inc., 1986. Pp. 391–398.

20. Patton, G. N., and Kistner, R. W. Surgery of the Oviduct. In *Atlas of Infertility Surgery* (2nd ed.). Boston: Little, Brown, 1984. Pp. 213–310.

21. Reed, T. P., and Erb, R. Hysteroscopic tubal occlusion with silicone rubber. *Obstet. Gynecol.* 61:388, 1983.

22. Schwimmer, M., et al. Postoperative hysterosalpingogram: radiographic-surgical correlation. *Radiology* 157:313, 1985.

23. Sheikh, H. H. Hysterosalpingographic follow-up of the partial salpingectomy type of sterilization. *Am. J. Obstet. Gynecol.* 128:858, 1977.

24. Spring, D. B. Fallopian tube occlusion rings: A consideration in the differential diagnosis of ureteral calculi. *Radiology* 145:51, 1982.

25. Vasquez, G., Winston, R. M. L., and Brosens, I. A. Tubal mucosa and ectopic pregnancy. *Br. J. Obstet. Gynaecol.* 90:468, 1983.

26. Winfield, A. C., and Wentz, A. C. *Diagnostic Imaging of Infertility.* Baltimore: Williams & Wilkins, 1987. Pp. 127–157.

27. Winston, R. M. L. Progress in tubal surgery. *Clin. Obstet. Gynaecol.* 8:653, 1981.

28. Yoon, I., and Poliakoff, S. R. Laparoscopic tubal ligation. A follow-up report on the Yoon falope ring methodology. *J. Reprod. Med.* 23:76, 1979.

Chapter 4
Diseases of the Uterus

Leiomyomas

Leiomyomas, or fibroids, are the most common tumors of the uterus [13]. Twenty percent of all women develop these benign nodules. Their incidence increases with age, and they are more frequent in black women than in white women. Myomas consist of smooth muscle, similar to myometrium, and varying amounts of fibrous tissue, arranged in a whorled pattern and surrounded by thin connective tissue, which allows easy surgical enucleation. They usually present as multiple discrete firm nodules varying in size from microscopic to enormous. The etiology of myomas is unclear, but it is well established that estrogen stimulates their growth. During pregnancy fibroids may increase markedly in size, whereas after menopause they stop growing and may regress. As leiomyomas increase in size they can outgrow their blood supply and undergo central ischemia and cystic degeneration. In older women the smooth muscle cells progressively atrophy and are replaced by fibrous tissue with a propensity to calcify. Malignant sarcomatous degeneration is very rare and occurs in 0.1 percent of leiomyomas [6].

Most leiomyomas originate within the myometrium of the body and fundus of the uterus. Infrequently they involve the uterine ligaments, lower uterine segment, and cervix. The majority are embedded within the myometrial wall in an intramural location. When they occur beneath the peritoneal covering of the uterus they are called subserosal. Myomas that elevate the endometrium and protrude into the uterine cavity are designated as submucosal (Fig. 4-1). Both subserosal and submucosal fibroids may become pedunculated. Although submucosal myomas are the least common they account for most clinical symptoms, including excessive menstrual bleeding, infertility, and spontaneous abortions. The mechanism of bleeding is unknown. Dilatation of the endometrial venous plexus or atrophy and ulceration of the endometrium overlying the mass may cause menorrhagia [6]. The mechanism of infertility is similarly obscure. Submucosal myomas may interfere with proper nutrition and function of the endometrium and prevent implantation or appropriate growth of a gestation [20]. Increased uterine contractility or abnormal blood flow to fetus may lead to recurrent miscarriages [6]. Obstruction of the fallopian tubes or cervix by myomas is rare.

The diagnostic approach to uterine leiomyomas is based primarily on the clinical situation. Pelvic ultrasound is always the initial study in the evaluation of a pelvic mass. In older women sonography is often followed by abdominal computed tomography to stage uterine or ovarian malignancy. In the younger patient and especially when myomectomy is planned to preserve childbearing capacity, a hysterosalpingogram is needed to determine the relationship of the myoma to the uterine cavity. Hysterosalpingography is also recommended when a myoma is suspected in a young woman with abnormal uterine bleeding, infertility, or recurrent abortion.

Fig. 4-1. Illustration of uterine myomas. A. Submucosal. B. Intramural. C. Subserosal. The size and position of a leiomyoma determine the severity of uterine cavity distortion.

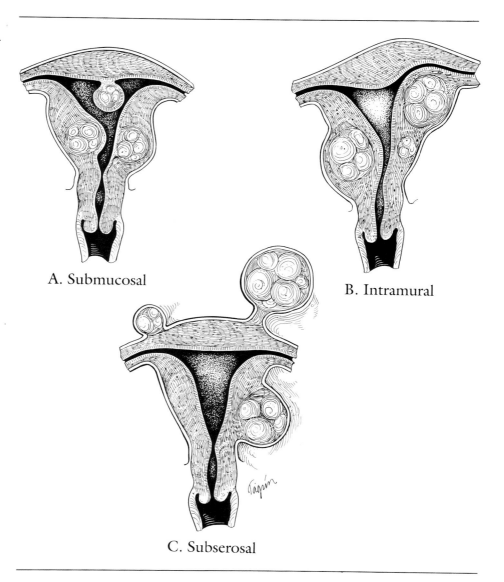

A. Submucosal

B. Intramural

C. Subserosal

Hysterosalpingography

Unless calcified, leiomyomas are detected during hysterosalpingography only to the extent that they enlarge and distort the cavity of the uterus. Subserosal myomas may be inapparent (Fig. 4-2) unless they are large enough to cause obvious displacement of the uterus. Intramural myomas deform the shape of the uterine cavity according to their size and location (Fig. 4-3). Submucosal myomas produce a filling defect within the uterine cavity and are quite easily seen as contrast first enters the uterus (Fig. 4-4).

Fig. 4-2. Serosal my-
omas. A. Plain film of
the pelvis shows multi-
ple calcified leiomyomas
(*arrows*). The patient
was a young woman
who recently had a nor-
mal delivery. During
pregnancy an ultrasound
had detected a very
abnormal uterine
configuration. B. Hys-
terosalpingogram con-
firmed the serosal loca-
tion of most of the
myomas (*arrows*) with
no distortion of the
uterine cavity. (Courtesy
of Dr. Patricia Fogel-
man, Colorado Springs,
Colo.)

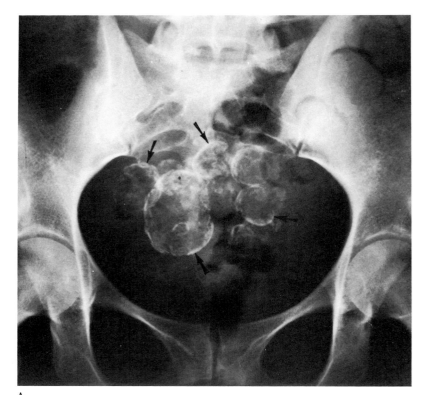

A

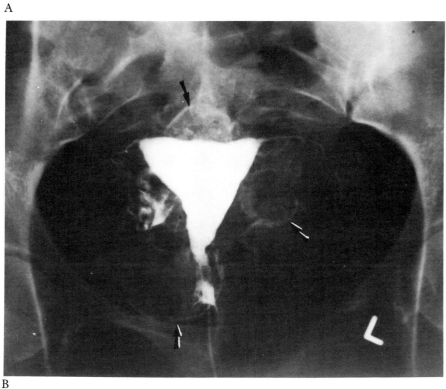

B

Fig. 4-3. Intramural myoma. A. Plain film of the pelvis shows displacement of the intrauterine balloon catheter toward the right side. The patient was a 30-year-old woman with infertility and a pelvic mass. B. Hysterosalpingogram demonstrated displacement of the uterus toward the right by a mass within the left wall of the uterus. The mass caused a smooth elongation of the left side of the uterine cavity and elevation of the left fallopian tube (*arrows*). The tubes were otherwise normal. Myomectomy removed an 8-cm left transmural myoma. The patient delivered a normal infant 18 months after surgery.

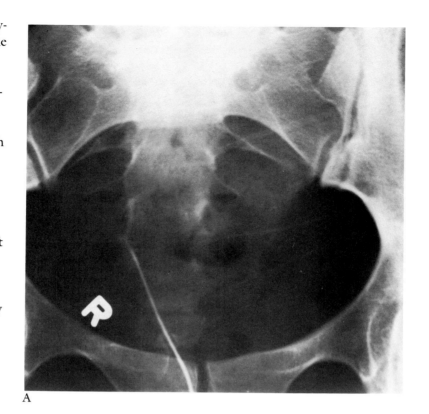

A

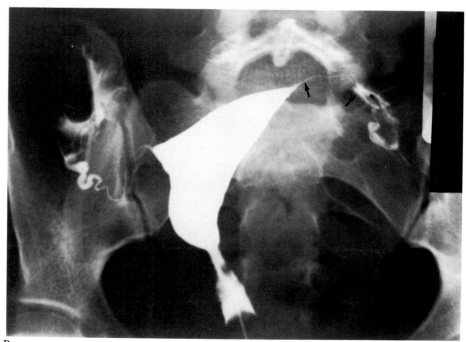

B

Fig. 4-4. Submucosal myoma. A 32-year-old woman underwent a hysterosalpingogram after an unsuccessful attempt to remove a Copper-7 IUD. A. Early filling of the uterine cavity showed the IUD (*open arrow*) displaced by a large submucosal filling defect (*closed arrows*). B. Larger amounts of contrast surrounded the IUD and the submucosal myoma. C. A total of 30 ml of contrast totally obscured the contents of the uterine cavity. The fallopian tubes were dilated and obstructed. At surgery an intracavitary IUD and a 7.5-cm submucosal myoma were removed. Bilateral hydrosalpinx required tubal reconstruction.

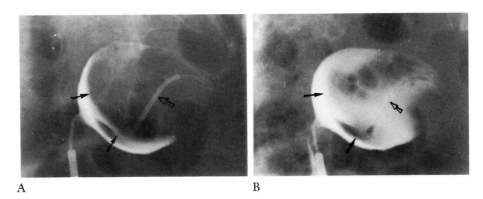

A   B

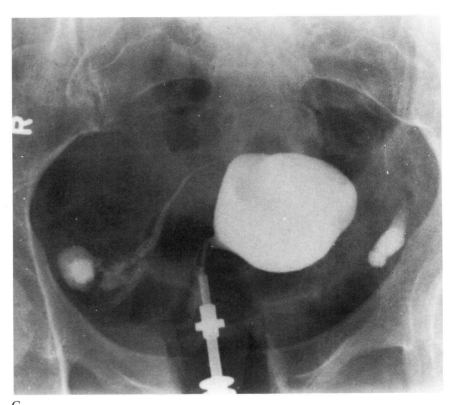

C

The filling defect may be obscured by subsequent introduction of larger quantities of contrast. Small filling defects must be differentiated from air bubbles, endometrial polyps, blood clots, and retained products of conception. Air bubbles are promptly displaced and flushed out of the tubes by tilting the head of the radiographic table upward and introducing more contrast. Endometrial polyps are more likely to be multiple and are smaller and more sharply outlined than submucosal fibroids, while blood clots and retained placenta have more angular outlines (Fig. 4-5). A large smooth filling defect may present an appearance that is completely indistinguishable from that of an intrauterine pregnancy (Fig. 4-6).

Fig. 4-5. Hysterosalpin-
gogram in a 35-year-old
woman 1 month follow-
ing a first trimester miscarriage. Retained prod-
ucts of conception are
seen as irregular filling
defects within the right
uterine horn (*arrows*).

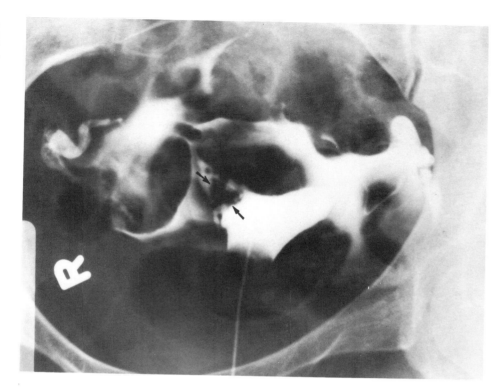

Fig. 4-6. Teaching col-
lection hysterosalpingo-
gram performed in 1940
demonstrates a 3-month
intrauterine pregnancy.
The patient subsequently
delivered a normal
infant.

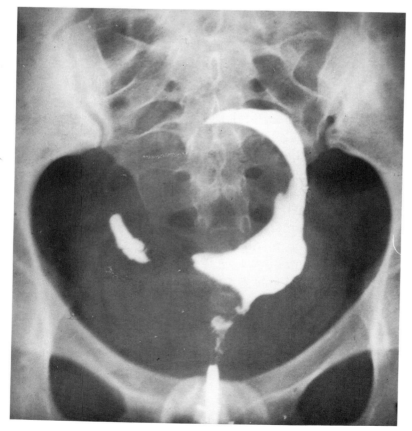

Fig. 4-7. Hysterosalpin-
gogram of a young
woman with infertility
and menorrhagia
showed a small sub-
mucosal myoma (*arrows*)
along the right uterine
wall. Hysteroscopic re-
moval was easily
achieved with a cysto-
scope-resectoscope.

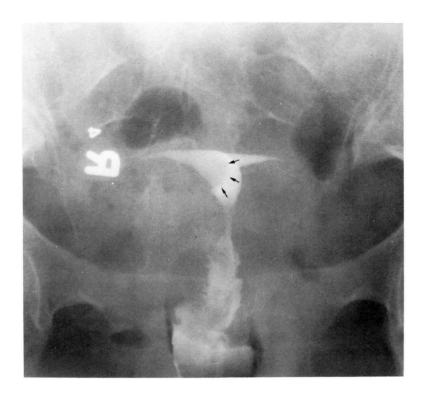

Both intramural and submucosal myomas may cause marked enlargement of the uterine cavity. The increase in size remains a mystery; it may be
caused by hypotony of the uterine muscle, or it may be secondary to actual
increased size of the uterus in response to the growing neoplasm [27].
The hysterosalpingogram may show an obviously enlarged and distorted
uterine cavity. When enlargement is only mild the volume of contrast
needed to fill the cavity provides an accurate gauge of size. Usually if more
than 6 cc of contrast is used before tubal filling is observed the uterus is
pathologically enlarged [27]. Uterine cavity enlargement is a very reliable
sign of the presence of a myoma but may not indicate its exact location
(anterior, posterior, fundus, or body) unless there is an accompanying
indentation of the wall or a filling defect. Lateral views and correlation with
ultrasound can further pinpoint the position of the myoma. Accurate localization is valuable to the surgeon who wants to keep uterine incisions to a
minimum during myomectomy and has a special interest in removing the
submucosal myomas responsible for most of the patient's symptoms. Hysteroscopic excision of small submucosal fibroids is an alternative to myomectomy [10] (Fig. 4-7). After myomectomy, hysterosalpingography reveals that even a greatly distorted uterine cavity can return to normal [41]
(Fig. 4-8).

114   Diseases of the uterus

Fig. 4-8. A 39-year-old patient presented with primary infertility and sonographic diagnosis of fibroids. The patient had bilateral tuboplasties 13 years before the study. Hysterosalpingograms (A) pre- and (B) post-myomectomy. A. Fifty ml of contrast was needed to fill a rounded and markedly enlarged uterine cavity with a large submucosal filling defect along the right wall. Venous run-off (*open arrows*) was misinterpreted as normal fallopian tube filling. The balloon catheter (*arrow*) was in the uterine cavity. B. Repeat study 1 year after removal of a 6-cm submucosal myoma. Uterine cavity was normal in size and shape. There was venous intravasation of contrast (*arrows*) and both fallopian tubes demonstrated interstitial obstruction.

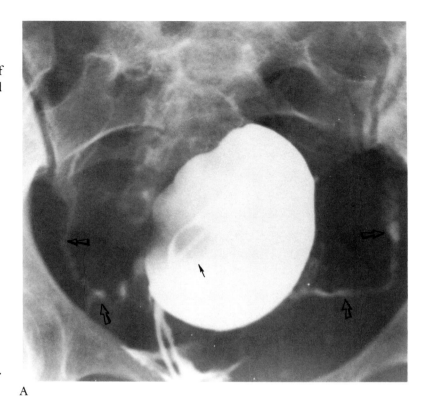

A

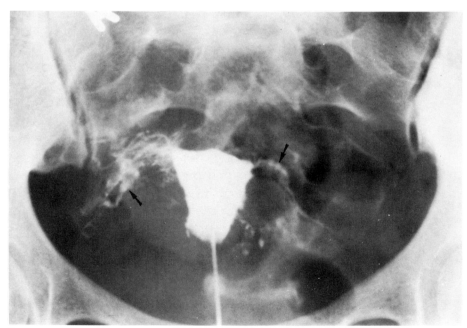

B

Fig 4-9. A 32-year-old patient with excessive bleeding and very prolonged menses. The hysterosalpingogram showed a huge submucosal myoma diffusely enlarging the uterine cavity (*arrows*). The right fallopian tube appeared normal, but not enough contrast was used to fill the left fallopian tube. The patient refused surgery.

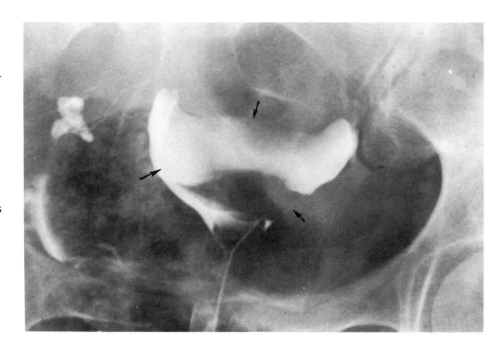

Submucosal myomas grow underneath the mucosal lining of the uterus and stretch the mucosa into a smooth surface over a filling defect of variable size. If the mass is large, there is simultaneous generalized enlargement of the uterine cavity (Fig. 4-9). If the myoma is small, there is localized enlargement of the area. For example, a uterine horn housing a small myoma becomes disproportionately larger than the contralateral horn (Fig. 4-10). Intramural fibroids, on the other hand, grow at variable distances from the uterine cavity. If large, they will indent and elongate one side of the uterine wall; and if near the cornua they may displace or stretch the fallopian tube (Fig. 4-11). Small intramural myomas produce more subtle changes in the configuration of the uterine cavity that makes them more difficult to find on the hysterosalpingogram. These changes include localized irregularity of the endometrium and localized straightening or asymmetry of the uterine wall. Small subserosal myomas may not be detected on hysterosalpingograms. However, as subserosal fibroids increase in size, they may produce obvious displacement of the uterus (Fig. 4-12). Pietila [27] correlated the roentgen and operative findings of 829 uterine myomas and found that the hysterosalpingogram identified 100 percent of submucosal, 73 percent of intramural, 62 percent of subserosal, and 86 percent of multiple fibroids. The roentgen report was correct on the average in 88 percent of cases and incorrect in 12 percent.

In the process of investigating the uterus for fibroids, it is crucial to carefully evaluate the fallopian tubes. A small minority of fibroids may be

Fig. 4-10. A. Oblique and (B) anteroposterior views of a hysterosalpingogram show a small submucosal myoma causing localized enlargement of the left uterine horn (*arrow*). (Courtesy of Dr. David Grant, New York, N.Y.)

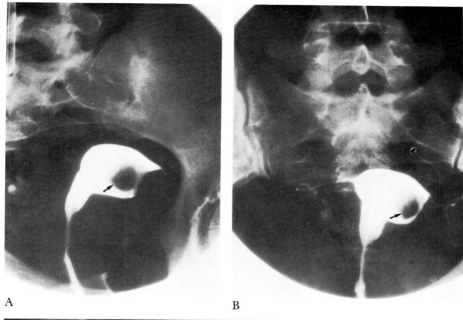

A   B

Fig. 4-11. A 25-year-old woman presented with menorrhagia and infertility. The hysterosalpingogram, using 12 ml of contrast, showed a rounded indentation along the left uterine wall (*arrows*) and draping of the left fallopian tube over the mass. At myomectomy an 8.5-cm left transmural myoma was removed. The fallopian tubes appeared normal.

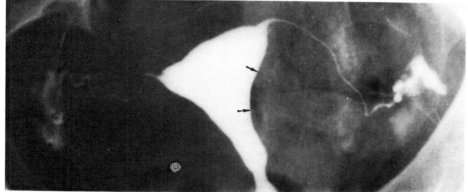

located near the cornua in a position that may cause fallopian tube obstruction (Fig. 4-13), but the great majority do not interfere with the mechanical passage of contrast into the tubes. Delayed opacification of the tubes may result from the large volume of contrast sometimes needed to fill the enlarged uterine cavity (Fig. 4-14); nevertheless the study is not complete until the tubes are well demonstrated. Simultaneous myomectomy and tuboplasty have a very low rate of subsequent successful pregnancy [30], but current microsurgical techniques may improve operative results in the future.

Fig. 4-12. A 35-year-old woman presented with bladder symptoms secondary to an enlarging pelvic mass. A. Film of the pelvis obtained during an intravenous urogram showed contrast in the bladder (*B*) and a large pelvic mass (*arrows*). B. The hysterosalpingogram showed marked anterior and superior displacement of the uterus and some straightening of the right uterine wall. Six serosal myomas were removed at surgery, the largest measuring 8 cm in diameter and fixed posteriorly to the cul-de-sac.

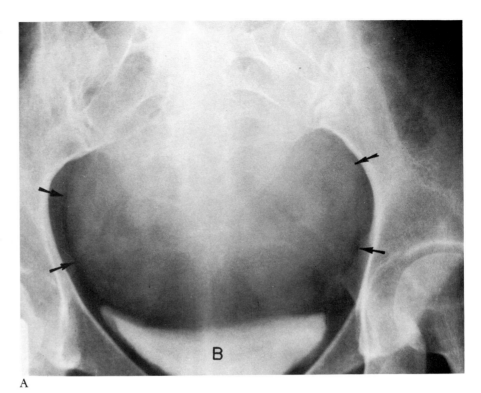

A

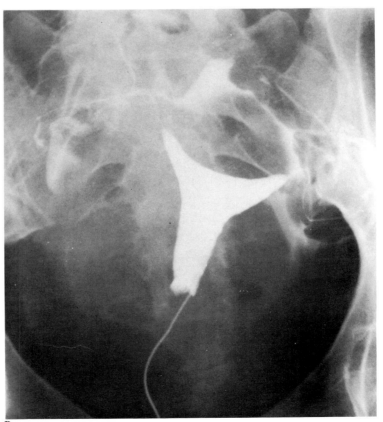

B

Fig. 4-13. Hysterosalpingogram in a 27-year-old woman with menorrhagia and anemia. A. Early filling film showed a rounded uterine cavity with a small submucosal filling defect in the area of the left horn (*arrow*). B. Later film, after the introduction of 30 ml of contrast, showed a persistent obstruction of the left fallopian tube. The right tube was normal. At surgery a single 9-cm submucosal and transmural myoma was removed from the left cornu.

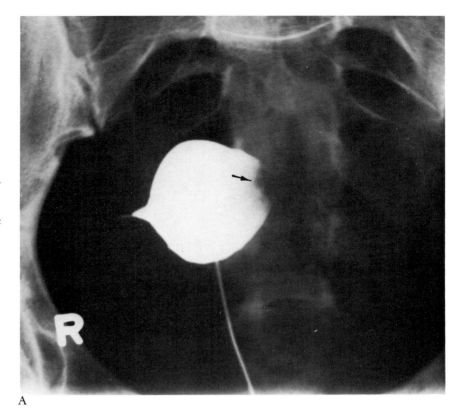

A

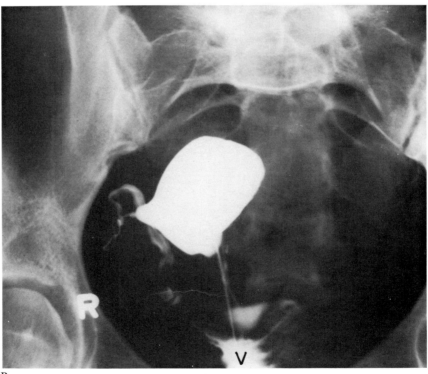

B

Fig. 4-14. Hysterosalpingograms before (A) and after (B) treatment of multiple fibroids with leuprolide acetate (GnRH analog). A. Initial hysterosalpingogram required 120 ml of contrast to fill an enormously enlarged uterine cavity. The fallopian tubes are underfilled. B. After 6 months of hormonal treatment the uterine cavity has decreased in size, requiring only 40 ml of contrast for adequate display of a rounded cavity and normal fallopian tubes. Magnetic resonance imaging of the uterus was performed at the time of the second hysterosalpingogram and demonstrated multiple submucosal, intramural, and subserosal fibroids. At myomectomy 14 nodules were removed, ranging from 0.7 to 6.5 cm in diameter. (Courtesy of Dr. Susan Stafford, Boston, Mass.)

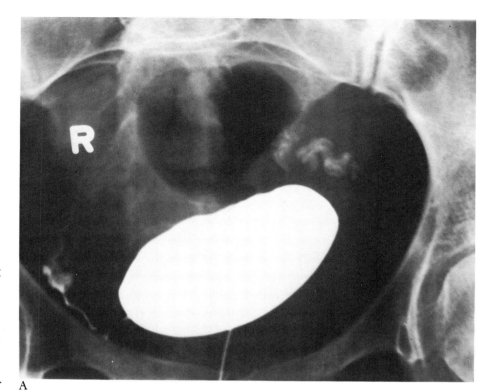

A

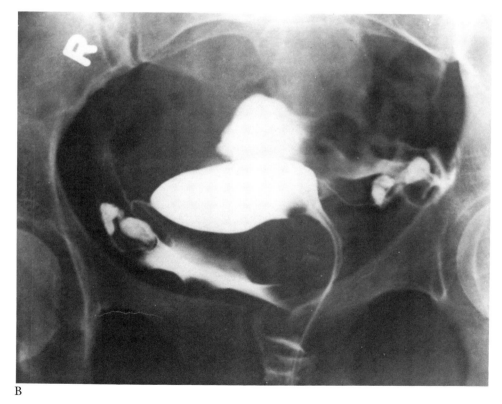

B

Ultrasound

Pelvic ultrasound and hysterosalpingography offer complementary views of uterine myomas. On sonography the fibroid uterus usually appears large and lobulated [14] (Fig. 4-15). A mass may be evident, with its echo texture only slightly altered from that of normal myometrium. Central degeneration will permit thorough transmission of the sound beam and give the mass a cystic appearance and a sharp back wall, whereas large amounts of fibrous tissue will attenuate sound transmission and obscure the back wall of the mass [15] (Fig. 4-16). Calcification produces sharp acoustic shadows. Sonography allows determination of uterine size and easy evaluation of the rate of tumor growth. Rapidly growing uterine myomas have been described in anovulatory patients secondary to prolonged unopposed estrogen stimulation [35]. Ultrasound is ideal to monitor the growth and position of fibroids during pregnancy. If a myoma is in contact with the placenta the patient is more prone to complications such as spontaneous abortion, premature labor, and postpartum hemorrhage [42]. Rapid growth of a myoma in a postmenopausal woman suggests sarcomatous degeneration.

A retroverted uterus may be mistaken for a myomatous uterus on ultrasound because the posteriorly located fundus appears large and hypoechoic and simulates a myoma or other solid mass [1]. Pedunculated myomas also present difficulties in sonographic diagnosis. Unless the attachment to the uterus is identified, a pedunculated subserosal fibroid may erroneously be called an adnexal mass, especially if cystic degeneration simulates a cystic ovary. A degenerated pedunculated submucosal fibroid may resemble an incomplete abortion (Fig. 4-17). Prolapse of a submucosal myoma may be demonstrated on serial ultrasound as an echogenic mass seen at one time below the cervix and at another time within the endometrial cavity [40].

In summary, pelvic ultrasound provides a reliable screening tool for the diagnosis and characterization of uterine myomas. Leiomyomas often distort the uterus and render it difficult to locate the endometrial cavity on sonography. Hysterosalpingography provides a specific demonstration of the structural changes exerted by a myoma on the uterine cavity.

Fig. 4-15. Uterine fibroids. Pelvic ultrasound in a 30-year-old woman with infertility and a myomectomy 10 years before the study was performed. A. Sagittal view showed a diffusely enlarged and abnormally shaped uterus. B. Transverse view showed a large lobulated uterus. The echo texture of the fibroids was similar to that of normal myometrium. The endometrial cavity could not be identified. Hysterectomy revealed a uterus enlarged by innumerable tan, whorled leiomyomas varying in size from 2 mm to 2 cm in serosal, intramural, and submucosal positions.

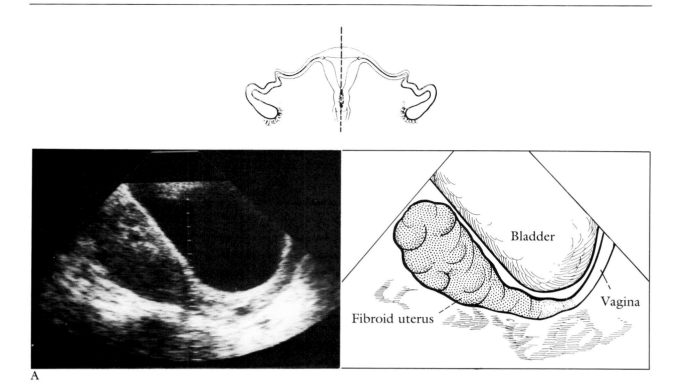

A

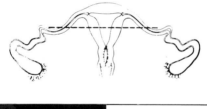

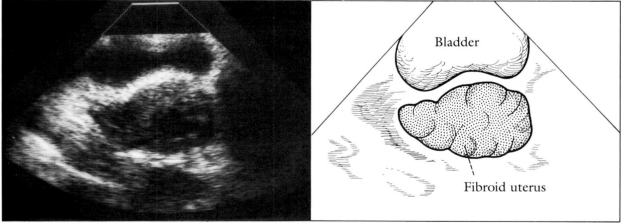

B

Fig. 4-16. Uterine fibroid and ovarian cyst. Pelvic ultrasound in a 29-year-old woman with a pelvic mass. A. Sagittal view shows two masses. The inferior mass is a diffusely enlarged echogenic uterus; the superior mass is a cystic ovarian mass separate from the uterus.

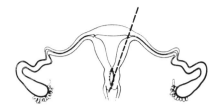

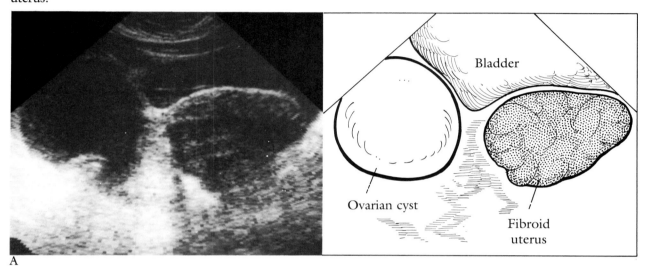

A

B. Transverse view at level of the left ovary shows a cystic mass with a sharp back wall and good thorough transmission of the ultrasound beam.

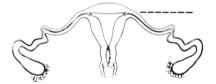

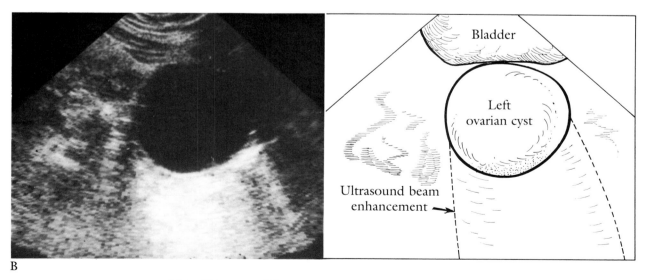

B

Fig. 4-16 (cont.) C. Midline transverse view shows an echogenic mass in the posterior uterus with no sharp back wall and attenuation of the sound beam. Surgery revealed a 9-cm left ovarian cystadenoma and an 8-cm posterior uterine myoma with a uniform fibrous center.

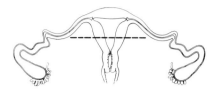

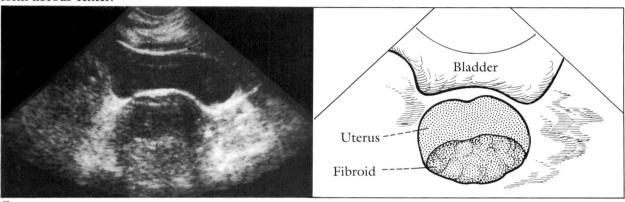

C

Fig. 4-17. A 40-year-old patient presented with 7 years of infertility and recent severe dysmenorrhea and menor-

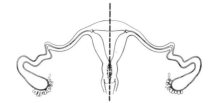

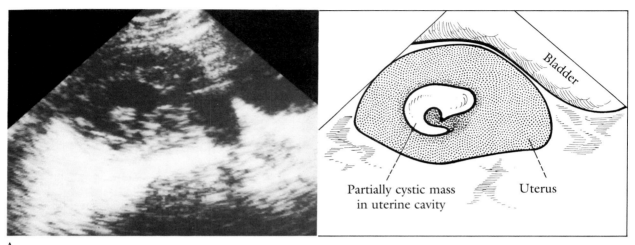

Bladder

Partially cystic mass
in uterine cavity

Uterus

A

rhagia. A. Sagittal ultrasound of the pelvis shows an enlarged uterus with a central lucent cavity. The appearance suggests an incomplete abortion. Curettage revealed fragments of smooth muscle tumor and no evidence of trophoblastic tissue. B and C. Early and late filling views of the hysterosalpingogram show an enlarged cervical canal and fundus. There is a large rounded submucous fundal defect (*closed arrows*).

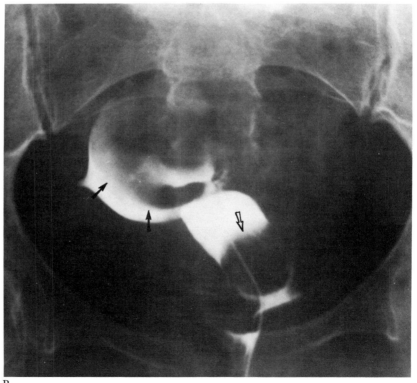

B

Fig. 4-17 (cont.) Tubal filling was never achieved because of vaginal (*V*) reflux. The balloon catheter (*open arrow*) was inflated with 7 ml of water. At surgery a 9.5 cm submucosal pedunculated fundal myoma with extensive cystic degeneration was removed. The patient delivered a normal infant 18 months after myomectomy.

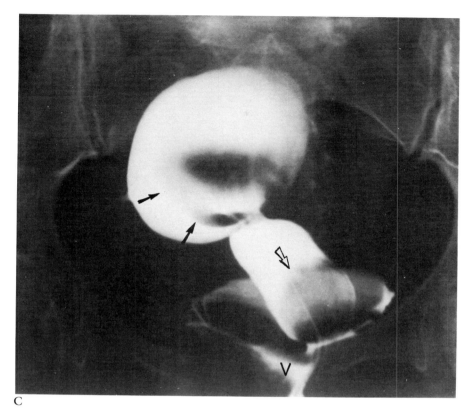

C

Endometrial Lesions

Diverse endometrial lesions are encountered while delineating the uterine cavity with contrast. This is especially true when the indication for hysterosalpingography is abnormal uterine bleeding. Asymptomatic endometrial lesions are also often found incidentally during infertility evaluation. This section describes the appearance and significance of uterine cavity lesions such as polyps, endometrial hyperplasia, endometrial carcinoma, and adenomyosis.

Endometrial Polyps

Endometrial polyps consist of endometrial tissue attached to the mucosa by a stalk. Polyps measure between 0.5 and 3.0 cm in diameter, may be single or multiple, and may appear before or after menopause [13]. The exact incidence of endometrial polyps is unknown, and they are often removed during curettage and not recognized. Polyps are likely to be entirely asymptomatic unless they protrude through the cervix or ulcerative changes in the endometrium cause abnormal bleeding. The great majority of polyps are benign, but in the postmenopausal woman they must be regarded with some suspicion because 10 to 15 percent may be associated with malignancy [18]. Only 1 percent of polyps undergo malignant degeneration. The treatment of polyps consists of hysteroscopic excision followed by curettage to remove any other remaining small polyps [10].

127

Fig. 4-18. Endometrial polyps (*arrows*) visible on hysterosalpingogram. (Courtesy of Dr. David Grant, New York, N.Y.)

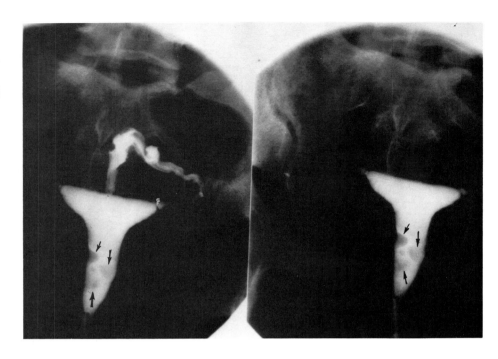

Hysterosalpingography. On hysterography polyps appear as small, rounded, sharply demarcated intrauterine filling defects (Fig. 4-18). They are easily obscured by contrast (Fig. 4-19). To evaluate them a second time, the contrast can be suctioned out of the uterus at the end of the study. Unlike evacuation, gradual removal of contrast through the Foley catheter allows better control of the optimal volume needed to visualize small cavitary defects. Suction may also remove small amounts of mucus or blood, which can mimic polyps. Air bubbles are a common source of error and must be carefully flushed out of the cavity. Submucosal myomas may present differential difficulties, but they usually enlarge the uterine cavity while polyps seldom do (Fig. 4-20). The radiologic image is an excellent guide to the hysteroscopic removal of polyps [10].

Fig. 4-19. Endometrial
polyp. Hysterosalpin-
gogram in a 25-year-old
with metrorrhagia.
A. Sequential spot films
during uterine filling
showed a lobulated
polyp (*arrow*) within the
lower uterine segment.
B. Final film demon-
strated the polyp (*arrow*)
less clearly because it is
obscured by contrast.

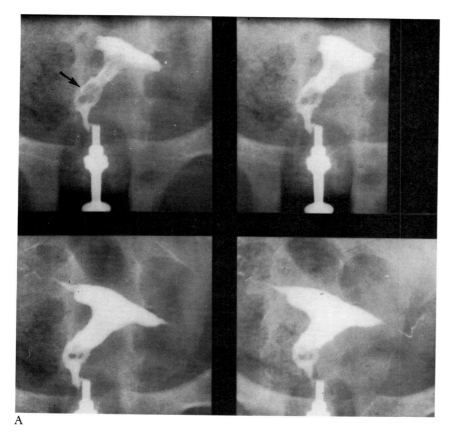

A

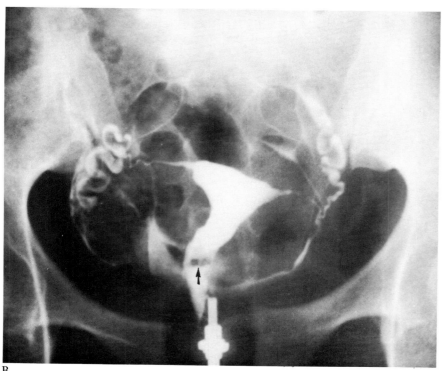

B

Fig. 4-20. Endometrial polyps. Hysterosalpingogram shows a minimally enlarged uterine cavity filled with multiple rounded uterine polyps (*arrows*). (Courtesy of Drs. H. Tristant and M. Benmussa, Paris, France.)

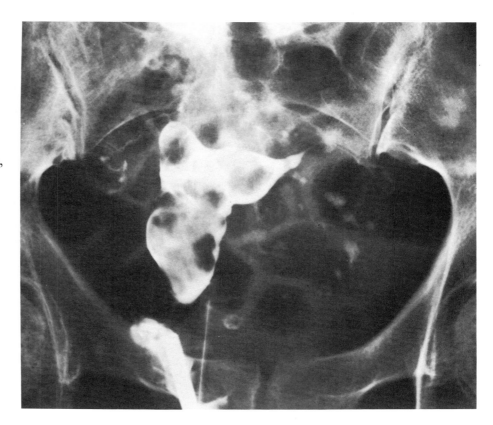

Endometrial Hyperplasia

Endometrial hyperplasia is a common cause of dysfunctional bleeding in pre- and postmenopausal women. In both groups the condition is produced by unimpeded estrogenic stimulation of the endometrium in the absence of progesterone [17]. During the menstrual years endometrial hyperplasia is associated with anovulatory cycles, in which a follicle fails to rupture and continues to produce estrogen with pronounced stimulation of the endometrium. These younger patients exhibit a mild form of hyperplasia, more often cystic, which regresses spontaneously after treatment. In the postmenopausal woman, hyperplasia may result from exogenous estrogen therapy or endogenous estrogen not produced by the ovary but by the conversion of the adrenal hormone androstenedione to estrone in the adipose tissues [17]. These older patients exhibit a severe adenomatous form of hyperplasia that frequently coexists with endometrial carcinoma.

Hysterosalpingography. On hysterography endometrial hyperplasia is characterized by a diffuse fine nodular (Fig. 4-21) or polypoid (Fig. 4-22) irregularity of the endometrial mucosa. The nodular defects vary in size from several millimeters to a centimeter. Very early underfilled films of the uterus are essential, since large volumes of contrast completely obliterate

Fig. 4-21. Endometrial hyperplasia. Hysterosalpingogram shows a fine nodular irregularity of the entire endometrial cavity. The endometrial hyperplasia was responsive to progesterone treatment. (Courtesy of Drs. H. Tristant and M. Benmussa, Paris, France.)

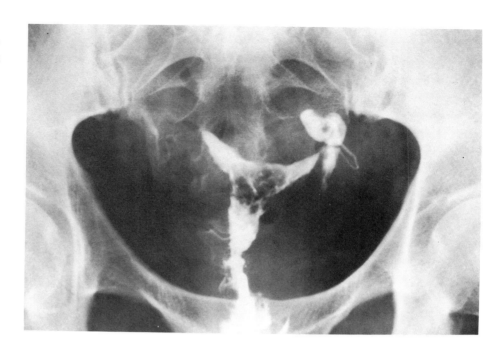

Fig. 4-22. Endometrial hyperplasia. Hysterosalpingogram shows a coarse polypoid irregularity of the entire endometrial mucosa. Hysterectomy confirmed diffuse endometrial hyperplasia. (Courtesy of the Department of Radiology, University of New Mexico Hospital, Albuquerque, N. Mex.)

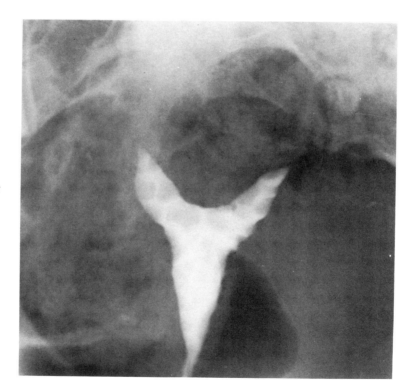

131

Fig. 4-23. A 27-year-old woman with infertility. The hysterosalpingogram was performed during the twenty-third day of the menstrual cycle and shows a thick and prominent but normal proliferative endometrium.

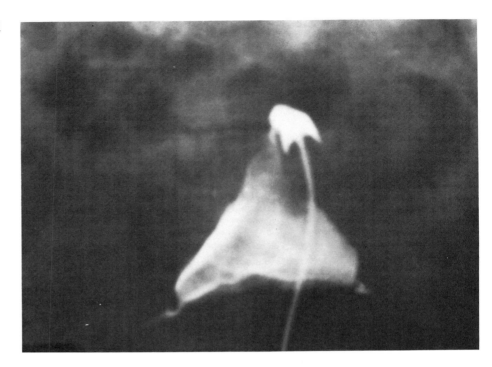

Fig. 4-24. Hysterosalpingogram in a young woman with infertility. Multiple longitudinal myometrial folds (*arrows*) are seen within the uterine cavity. Exact etiology is unknown; hysteroscopy was not performed.

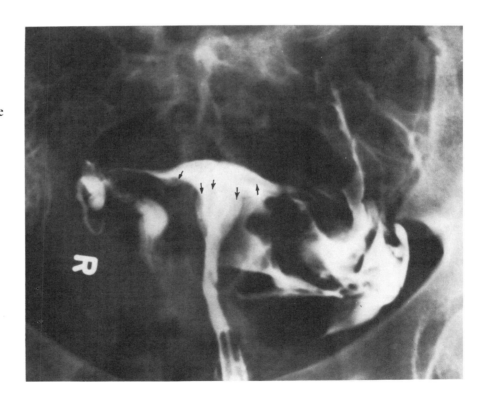

the mucosal pattern [37]. Although characteristic, the hysterographic appearance does not allow histologic differentiation between cystic and adenomatous hyperplasia. Hysterograms performed during the secretory phase of the menstrual cycle demonstrate a very prominent mucosal pattern (Fig. 4-23), which should not be confused with endometrial hyperplasia. Other sources of misinterpretation include mucous secretions and blood clots within the uterine cavity. A small percentage of patients demonstrate broad longitudinal folds parallel to the uterine cavity (Fig. 4-24). They are not correlated with the thickness or hormonal phase of the endometrium, but represent myometrial folds that may be remnants of müllerian duct fusion during fetal development [34].

Endometrial Carcinoma

Endometrial carcinoma is the most common gynecologic malignancy in the United States [18]. Its ascendancy is secondary both to an increased number of cases of endometrial cancer and a concomitant decline in the incidence of cervical cancer. Typically 95 percent of uterine endometrial carcinomas are adenocarcinomas, and 95 percent occur after menopause [13]. Although the etiology is unknown, prolonged or exaggerated estrogen stimulation is a contributing factor. Endometrial carcinoma has been associated with estrogen replacement therapy use for menopause. Patients with estrogen-producing ovarian tumors and anovulatory patients, especially those with polycystic ovaries, also have an increased incidence of endometrial carcinoma.

Hysterosalpingography. Hysterosalpingography is not presently used routinely for the investigation of uterine malignancy, but it may occasionally reveal an endometrial carcinoma in a young patient. Thus it is important to recognize the hysterographic appearance of such tumors. In the 1950s Norman [24] in Sweden, and in the 1970s Tak and coworkers at the Tufts-New England Medical Center [36] in Boston used hysterosalpingography to examine large numbers of patients with endometrial carcinoma. The radiographic appearance of the tumor corresponds to the macroscopic appearance and may be localized or diffuse. The localized mass grows as an exophytic tumor encroaching into the uterine cavity (Fig. 4-25). Contrast surrounds a mass of variable size, often with ragged contours, less often with a smooth outline. As the tumor enlarges, it is more likely to invade the myometrium (Fig. 4-26). Diffuse carcinoma extensively infiltrates the mucosa, producing a very irregular, spiculated endometrial cavity (Fig. 4-27).

The differential diagnosis includes large polyps for the smooth masses and severe endometrial hyperplasia for the infiltrative tumors. Both polyps and hyperplasia usually have a less aggressive appearance than carcinoma, and both also necessitate hysteroscopy or diagnostic curettage. The spread of malignant cells into the peritoneum during hysterography has never been documented and is probably less likely to occur than during surgical curettage.

Fig. 4-25. Endometrial carcinoma. Hysterosalpingogram in a 31-year-old infertile patient with an additional history of two episodes of spotting dark blood between menses. Multiple round filling defects (*arrows*) are seen within the uterine fundus. Endometrial carcinoma was diagnosed on curettage with no residual tumor found on hysterectomy specimen.

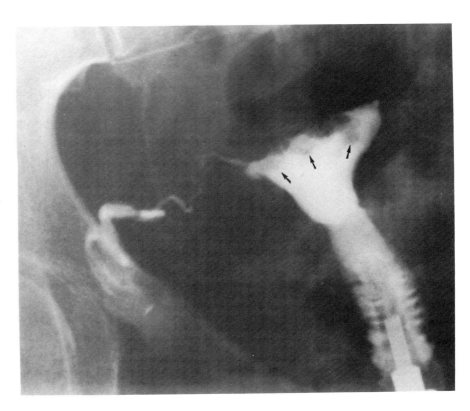

Fig. 4-26. Endometrial carcinoma. Hysterosalpingogram shows rounded irregular masses extending into the uterine cavity along the right wall and the fundus. Diffuse carcinoma of the endometrium infiltrating into the myometrium was found at surgery. (Courtesy of Drs. H. Tristant and M. Benmussa, Paris, France.)

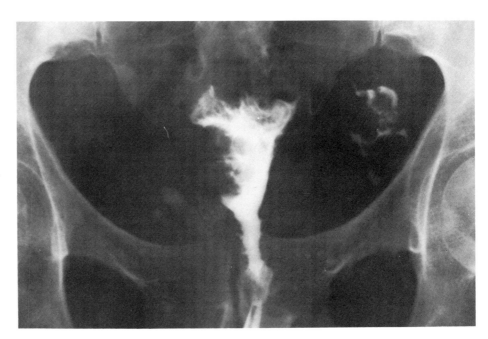

Fig. 4-27. Endometrial carcinoma. The hysterosalpingogram in a 57-year-old woman demonstrates a round mass within the left uterine horn (*arrow*) and a diffuse spiculated border of the entire uterine cavity. A carcinoma of the endometrium is present with diffuse involvement of the endometrial cavity. (Courtesy of Drs. H. Tristant and M. Benmussa, Paris, France.)

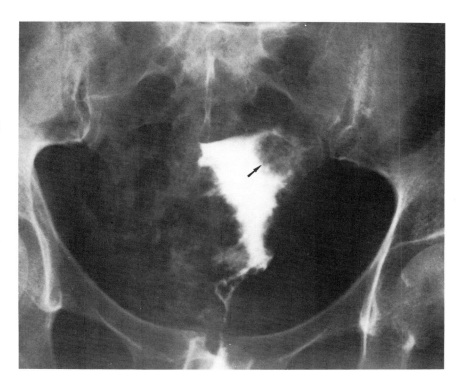

Adenomyosis

Adenomyosis refers to the presence of endometrium deep within the myometrial layer of the uterine wall. Sometimes it is called endometriosis interna to distinguish it from endometriosis externa or pelvic endometriosis. Adenomyosis usually occurs in the 40-year-old, parous woman, while endometriosis affects the younger, infertile patient [25]. In adenomyosis there is a growth of superficial endometrium deep into the underlying muscle with accompanying hyperplasia of the myometrium around the implants. There may be continuity of the glands with the surface endometrium or the muscle overgrowth may nip off the connection. The most frequent symptoms are menorrhagia and dysmenorrhea. The diagnosis is seldom suspected preoperatively, but routine examination of surgically excised uteri showed adenomyosis in 10 percent of specimens [26]. Adenomyoma is an encapsulated area of adenomyosis forming a discrete tumor nodule.

Hysterosalpingography. Hysterosalpingography is diagnostic of adenomyosis when short diverticular outpouchings extend outside the uterine cavity [22]. Most of the contrast-filled projections end in small sacs, less than 5 mm in diameter, and surround the cavity of the fundus and body of the uterus. The diverticuli may be localized to one area or involve the uterine wall diffusely. They are often short, shallow channels, but on occasion may become more complex and aborescent. The uterine cavity is usually normal in size or slightly enlarged. In a series studied by Marshak [22] only 25 percent of histologically proven cases of adenomyosis showed hysterog-

135

Fig. 4-28. Dilated cervi-
cal gland. Hysterosalpin-
gogram in a 35-year-old
woman with dysfunc-
tional bleeding shows
incidental filling of a dilated cervical gland (*arrow*). (V = vagina.)

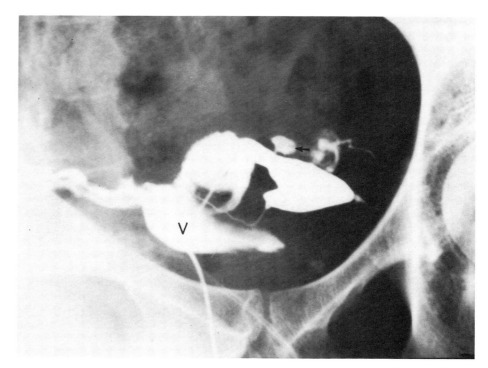

Fig. 4-29. Adenomy-
oma. A 33-year-old
woman presented with
infertility and menor-
rhagia. A. Hysterosal-
pingogram showed lo-
calized intravasation of
contrast into a round
mass (*arrows*) within the
wall of the endocervical
canal. B. Transverse and
(C) sagittal views of
the pelvic ultrasound
showed an echogenic
mass in the endocervix
resembling a fibroid. A
3-cm mass was easily
enucleated from the
right wall of the en-
docervix and proved to
be an adenomyoma.

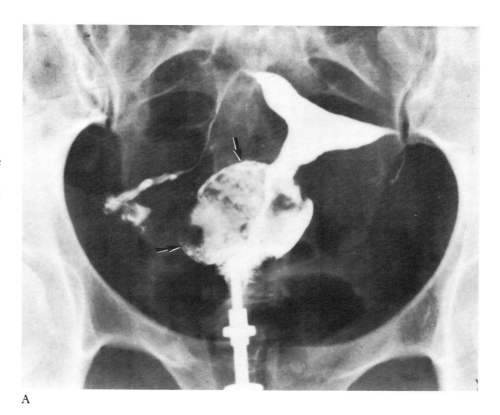

A

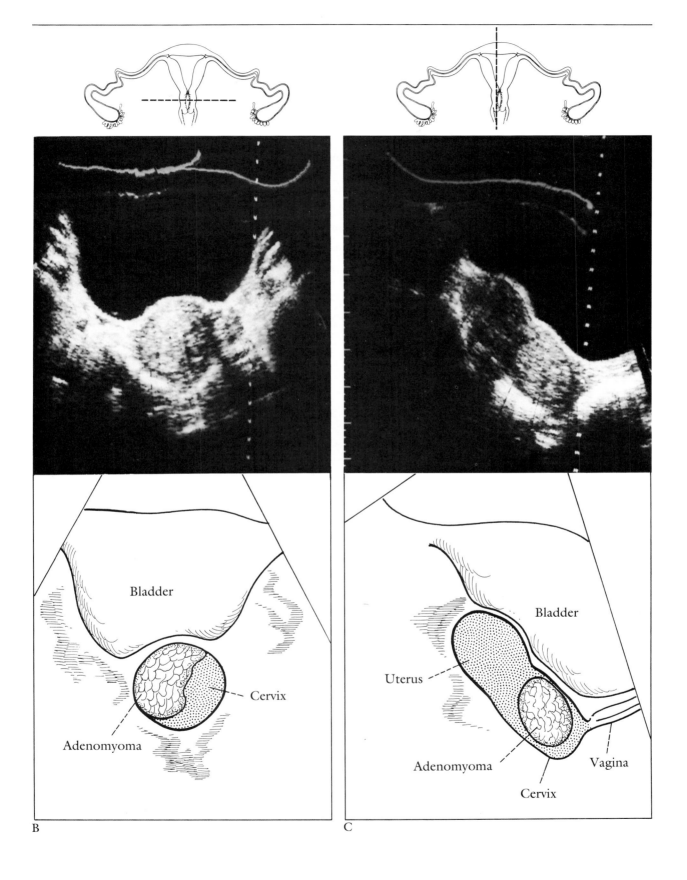

B

C

Bladder

Cervix

Adenomyoma

Uterus

Bladder

Adenomyoma

Cervix

Vagina

raphic abnormalities. The glandular elements may not fill because they lack continuity with the endometrium or because the communicating channel is blocked by secretions or blood. Cavities larger than 5 mm and those located in the endocervical canal are usually caused by dilated cervical glands (Fig. 4-28) and seldom due to adenomyosis [33]. The differential diagnosis includes localized intravasation of contrast into myometrial vascular channels, which is characterized by venous run-off, and endometrial hyperplasia, which may have a spiculated appearance, though the spicules remain confined entirely within the uterine cavity. The underlying overgrowth of the uterine muscle may produce a smooth filling defect in the uterine cavity resembling a submucosal fibroid. Very rarely contrast may demonstrate the glandular cavities contained within an adenomyoma (Fig. 4-29), though more commonly an adenomyoma cannot be differentiated from a fibroid.

Ultrasound of the Uterine Cavity

The normal sonographic appearance of the endometrial cavity is characterized by a thin echogenic line surrounded by an echo-poor zone [12]. The linear echo represents the endometrium and the echo-poor zone represents the vascular inner myometrial segment. Certain fluid collections within the endometrial cavity cause separation of the walls with an anechoic or relatively anechoic space between them. Menstrual blood, early or abnormal intrauterine pregnancy, pseudogestational sac, endometritis, and pyometra are all processes leading to echolucent accumulations [2]. Increased echogenicity within the endometrial cavity occurs either because of the presence of mucus, blood clot, retained products of conception, early hydatidiform mole, or foreign body (e.g., IUD), or secondary to abnormalities of the endometrium itself. Endometrial polyps, hyperplasia, and carcinoma give rise to increased endometrial echoes that are indistinguishable from each other [2].

Ultrasound is not an accurate method for detecting or staging carcinoma of the endometrium. Postmenopausal women with fluid-distended uterine cavities are often found to have carcinoma of the uterine corpus or cervix [5]. Pelvic sonography has been used with limited success in patients with histologically proven adenocarcinoma of the endometrium to determine the depth of myometrial invasion by tumor [12]. The introduction of endovaginal ultrasound promises to permit more accurate sonographic evaluation of endometrial lesions in the future.

The sonographic appearance of adenomyosis is very similar to that of leiomyomas. The uterus is generally enlarged, but it never attains the large size or lobulated contours seen with myomas. This enlargement is often localized to the posterior portion of the myometrium with anterior displacement of the endometrial cavity [4]. The endometrial glands may appear as irregular cystic spaces within the myometrium. If this appearance is seen with cystic and solid adnexal masses, the diagnosis of coexisting endometriosis, interna and externa, can be established [39].

Asherman's Syndrome: Intrauterine Adhesions

Intrauterine adhesions, or synechiae, usually result from vigorous curettage of the uterine cavity following obstetric delivery or abortion. During postpregnancy curettage, the basal layer of the endometrium is more easily denuded than at other times because the underlying myometrium is soft, and the "grating" sensation the surgeon feels when scraping the endometrium is lost [3]. The denuded endometrium then heals by forming single or multiple fibrous bands between the endometrial walls, which become partially or totally adherent to each other. Very rarely adhesions may form following a diagnostic curettage or some form of uterine surgery such as a myomectomy. In the 1950s Asherman popularized the syndrome complex caused by intrauterine adhesions and it now carries his name. The clinical manifestations of Asherman's syndrome include postcurettage amenorrhea or hypomenorrhea, infertility, and, to a lesser degree, dysmenorrhea [29]. When pregnancy does occur in these patients, it is fraught with the complications of recurrent abortion, premature labor, and placenta accreta or placenta previa. The exact incidence of uterine synechiae is unknown, but it is very likely that they are increasing in frequency because of increasing worldwide reliance on elective abortions for birth control.

Hysterosalpingography establishes the diagnosis and hysteroscopy confirms the presence of adhesions [21]. Under direct hysteroscopic control, the adhesions can be simply cut by the use of microscissors or diathermy. Following lysis of adhesions, an inflated Foley catheter or an IUD may be placed in the uterine cavity to prevent readherence of the cavity walls. Postoperative exogenous estrogens are often administered to promote endometrial epithelialization of the scarred surfaces. Successful restoration of the uterine cavity reestablishes normal menstruation, increases fertility, and decreases complications of pregnancy though it does not completely eliminate them.

Hysterosalpingography

Intrauterine adhesions have a characteristic appearance on hysterosalpingography but vary greatly in location and extent. Filling defects are usually seen within the uterine cavity that result from partial obliteration of the cavity at certain points where the anterior and posterior walls fuse. These points of adherence form "islands" around which the contrast flows [38]. The islands are sharply delineated; can be linear or triangular, single or multiple; and in general have angular contours (Fig. 4-30). Unlike other uterine cavity defects, increasing volumes of contrast will not completely obscure adhesions because there is no contrast flowing in front of or behind them (Fig. 4-31). Previous studies have shown that 65 percent of synechiae occur in the uterine fundus and body, while 35 percent occur in the endocervical canal [32]. Most adhesions are partial and allow intrauterine introduction of contrast for diagnosis. Occasionally synechiae may obliterate the entire endometrial cavity or obstruct the lower uterine segment and permit contrast opacification of only a short segment of blunt-ending cervical canal (Fig. 4-32). This situation may require the use of the vacuum

Fig. 4-30. Intrauterine adhesions. A 42-year-old woman presented with oligomenorrhea since a miscarriage and curettage 1 year before the study was performed. The hysterosalpingogram showed several linear and triangular adhesions within the uterine cavity (*arrows*). Multiple uterine synechiae were broken up during a repeat curettage. (From D. A. Hall and I. C. Yoder, Radiology in the Diagnosis and Therapy of Female Infertility. In J. F. Simeone [ed.], *Coordinated Diagnostic Imaging*. New York: Churchill Livingstone, 1984. Reprinted with permission.)

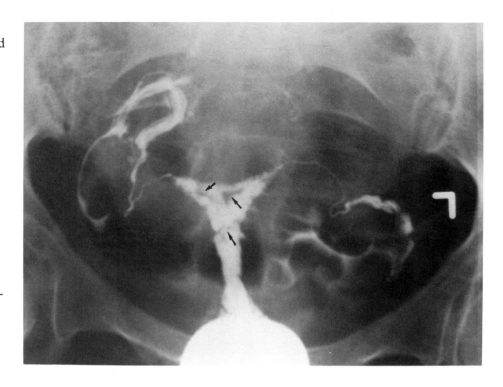

cannula since the Foley catheter will dislodge every time contrast increases the pressure within the obstructed endocervical canal. With the cannula in place, greater pressures can be generated and the persistent inability to introduce contrast into the uterine cavity will allow a confident diagnosis of adhesions. Hematometra does not occur despite obliteration of the endocervix because the remaining endometrium becomes refractory to hormonal stimulus [29].

March [21] has offered a simple hysteroscopic classification of intrauterine adhesions. It consists of three categories: mild, moderate, and severe; according to whether adhesions involve one-fourth, one-half, and three-fourths or more, respectively; of the uterine cavity. This is a useful classification because it is easy to remember and gives the clinician an approximate quantitative idea of the extent of the cavitary adhesions. It also allows a basis for comparison with postoperative hysterosalpingograms. Correlation between hysterosalpingography and hysteroscopy is excellent as long as two caveats are observed. First, hysteroscopy underestimates the severity of adhesions as seen on the radiographs, probably because the endoscopic technique itself causes disruption of some adhesions by forceful distension of the uterine cavity. Second, endometrial polyps and submucosal myomas may mimic intrauterine adhesions, but the former tend to have more rounded contours and are more easily obscured by contrast than the latter.

Fig. 4-31. Intrauterine adhesions. Hysterosalpingogram shows sharply demarcated intrauterine adhesions (*arrows*). A large volume of contrast does not obscure the adhesions. (Courtesy of Dr. Alan C. Winfield, Nashville, Tenn.)

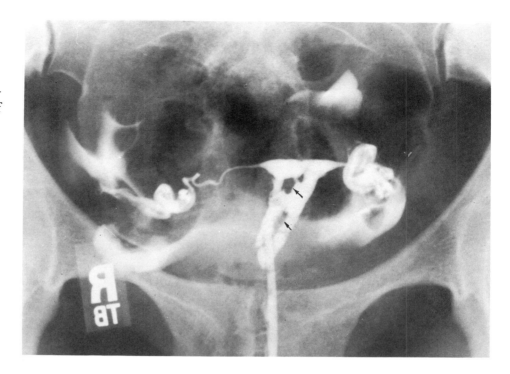

Fig. 4-32. A 28-year-old woman who had been amenorrheic since a therapeutic abortion 1 year before the study was performed. Hysterosalpingogram filled only the endocervical canal as the remainder of the endometrial cavity was obliterated by uterine synechiae.

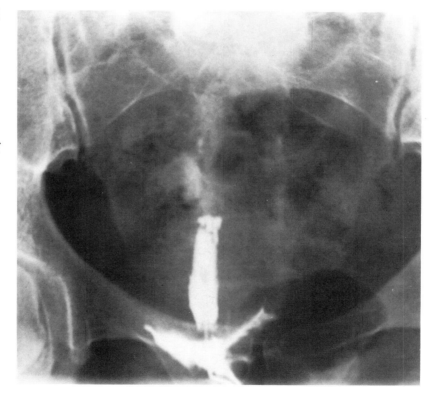

Fig. 4-33. Hysterosalpingogram demonstrates scarring and irregular contraction of the uterine cavity secondary to tuberculous endometritis. The fallopian tubes also show tuberculous changes with widening and obstruction of both isthmic segments. (Courtesy of Drs. H. Tristant and M. Benmussa, Paris, France.)

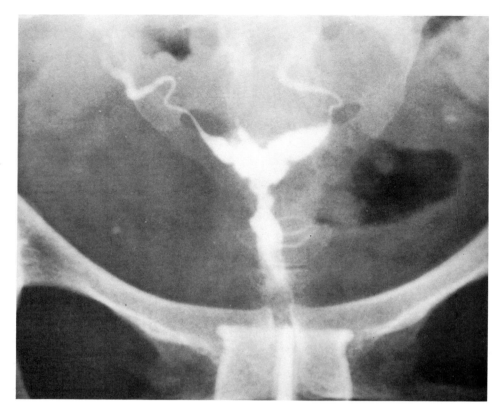

Fig. 4-34. A 32-year-old woman whose last menstrual period was 1 month ago prior to the study and whose pregnancy test was negative. The hysterosalpingogram showed a mildly enlarged uterine cavity with a double contour (*arrows*). A second pregnancy test was positive. The patient delivered a normal infant 8 months later.

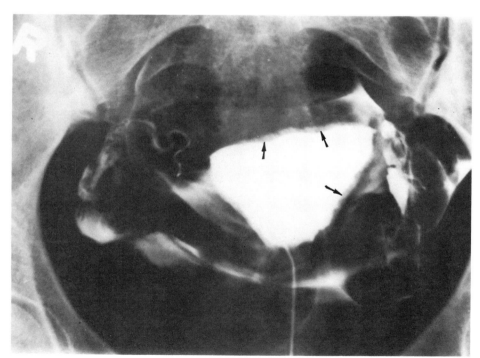

Tuberculous endometritis can cause marked scarring and contraction of the uterine cavity (Fig. 4-33). In such cases the amenorrhea is primary instead of secondary, and the tubes also demonstrate tuberculous changes [29]. Abnormal widening of the internal cervical os is sometimes associated with intrauterine adhesions.

Ultrasound

On ultrasound intrauterine adhesions are seen as very echogenic, asymmetric lines within the endometrial cavity [8]. The echogenic lines disappear after lysis of the adhesions.

Intrauterine Pregnancy

Inadvertent study of a pregnant uterus is almost inevitable in a busy radiology department doing a large number of hysterosalpingograms. The radiologist may neglect to verify menstrual dates; the patient may not realize she is pregnant because she has had vaginal bleeding resembling menses; or the pregnancy test may erroneously be reported as negative. Within the first few weeks after conception, a double-outlined uterine cavity is the earliest specific evidence of pregnancy [16]. A thin line of contrast surrounds the walls of the uterine cavity as contrast is introduced, giving the appearance of a double contour (Fig. 4-34). The line is produced by contrast underneath the decidual lining of the uterine cavity. The contrast does not penetrate into the myometrial vessels, as evidenced by the lack of venous opacification. A double contour is a normal finding in patients having hysterosalpingograms in the late secretory phase of the menstrual cycle [16]. The absence of a double outline does not exclude a very early intrauterine pregnancy, which may present as a nonspecific slight enlargement of the uterine cavity with nondistinct or fuzzy walls. By 3 to 4 weeks after conception a gestational sac becomes evident as a smooth intrauterine filling defect, which, when accompanied by a double contour, presents pathognomonic signs of pregnancy (Fig. 4-35). The hysterosalpingogram will not cause mechanical disruption of the pregnancy and seldom leads to abortion of the fetus.

As the pregnancy progresses the gestational sac presents as a large intrauterine filling defect, difficult to distinguish from a submucosal myoma except by history or by ultrasound examination (Fig. 4-36).

Fig. 4-35. A 31-year-old woman was admitted for myomectomy. Hysterosalpingogram was performed although she had skipped a period because a pregnancy test was (erroneously) reported as negative. A and B. Early filling views show a prominent endometrium consistent with decidual reaction. There is also a double uterine contour and an early gestational sac (*arrow*). C. The introduction of more contrast obscures the gestational sac and the decidual reaction but emphasizes the double contour (*arrows*). Curettage yielded placental tissue.

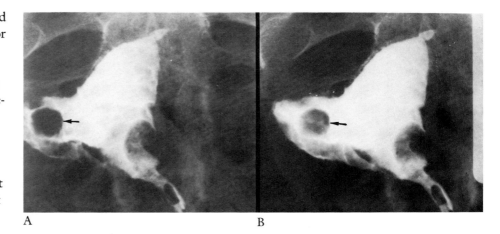

A   B

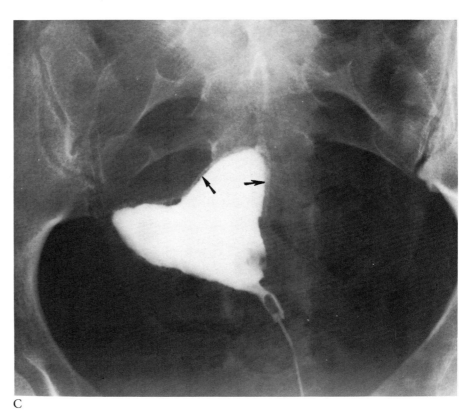

C

Fig. 4-36. Pregnancy. Hysterosalpingogram shows (A) a smooth rounded gestational sac and a double uterine contour. B. As more contrast was introduced the double contour was demonstrated better. Several air bubbles have been introduced into the uterine cavity with the contrast.

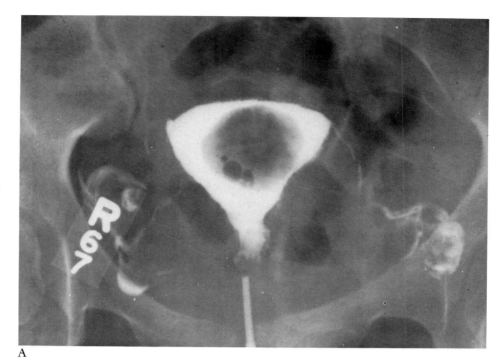

A

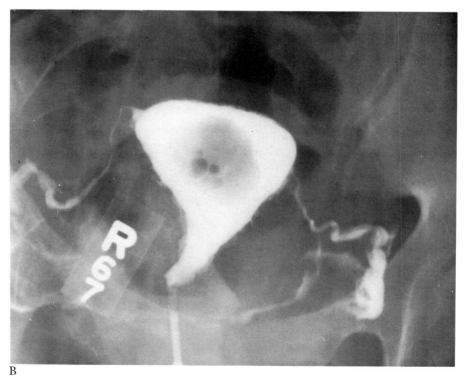

B

IUDs

In August 1985 the A. H. Robins Company filed for bankruptcy after 14,000 users of its Dalkon Shield IUD sought damages for pelvic infections and sterility. A few months later Ortho Pharmaceutical Corporation stopped selling its Lippes Loop, and early in 1986 G. D. Searle removed the Copper-7 and Tatum-7 IUDs from the market [11]. Ortho and Searle cited difficulties in obtaining liability insurance as reason for discontinuing the sale of IUDs in the United States even though their sale is approved by the Food and Drug Administration. The result is that Progestasert, a progesterone-releasing IUD, is the only IUD available in the United States.

The IUD is a highly effective reversible method of conception control, and its demise will probably increase the incidence of unwanted pregnancies and premature tubal sterilizations. Because of the association between IUD use and pelvic infection and the possibility of tubal infertility, the IUD is recommended mainly to parous women in their thirties [23]. It is estimated that 50 million women worldwide and 3 million American women use IUDs [31].

The exact mechanism by which an IUD prevents pregnancy is not known, but all IUDs cause a localized chronic endometritis which may interfere with implantation [7]. Pelvic pain and excessive menstrual bleeding are frequent side effects and the most common reason for elective removal of the IUD. Less frequent but more serious complications include spontaneous expulsion, uterine perforation, and pelvic infection. The expulsion rates vary between 2 and 15 percent, and are highest during the first few months of use and when the IUD is inserted less than 6 weeks postpartum [19]. Uterine perforation is uncommon and occurs in less than 1 per 1000 insertions. Perforation usually occurs at the time of insertion and is more strongly correlated to operator experience than to the type of IUD. The Copper-7 and Progestasert tend to perforate the uterine cervix, whereas Lippes Loop and Dalkon Shield more frequently perforate through the uterine body. Once an IUD is free in the peritoneal cavity, it presents the rare but serious risk of bowel obstruction caused by perforation or adhesions. Laparoscopic removal is usually easily accomplished. Epidemiologic studies suggest that there is an increased risk of acute pelvic infection among IUD users compared with that of nonusers, but the magnitude of the risk remains uncertain and is greatest for women with a previous history of pelvic infection or multiple sex partners, and for nulliparous women less than 25 years old [23]. The risk of primary tubal infertility appears to be significantly increased with the use of plastic IUDs, while marginally or not at all with copper-containing IUDs [9].

Radiology

Ultrasound is the principal radiologic method of assessing the intrauterine location of an IUD. The need arises most often when the IUD string can no longer be found in the vagina. The clinical possibilities include: IUD string lost or retracted into the uterine cavity, IUD expulsion, IUD perforation, and pregnancy. Sonography allows up to 100 percent localization of an intrauterine IUD. Lippes Loop and Copper-7 IUDs have type-specific morphology that allows their specific identification [7]. On longitudinal scans the Lippes Loop demonstrates four or five distinct high-amplitude endometrial cavity echoes (Fig. 4-37). The Copper-7 shows two distinct endometrial echoes, a short superior one and a long inferior echo caused by the long copper-wrapped limb (Fig. 4-38). IUDs also produce acoustic shadows, similar to those produced by renal stones and gallstones; entrance-exit reflections thought to represent echoes from the anterior and posterior surfaces of the IUD; and reverberation echoes, a trail of dense "comet tail" echoes sometimes seen with small metallic objects [2]. High-amplitude echoes and acoustic shadows may be caused by other intrauterine foreign bodies such as air, stents, and bones from an incomplete abortion. The IUD is normally found in a central position within the uterus; an eccentric position may indicate that it is embedded within the myometrium [28].

Fig. 4-37. A. Sagittal and (B) transverse sonograms of the pelvis demonstrate a Lippes Loop IUD centrally positioned within the uterine cavity.

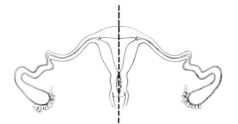

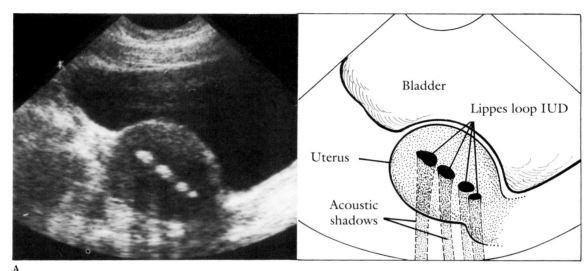

A

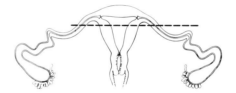

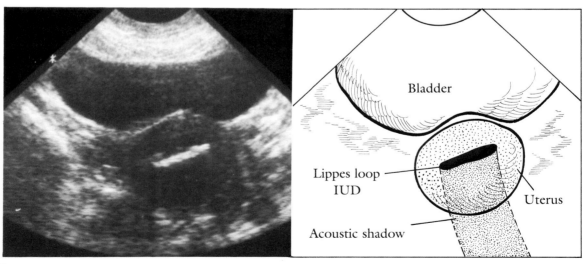

B

Fig. 4-38. A. Sagittal and (B) transverse sonograms of the pelvis show a Copper-7 IUD within the uterine cavity.

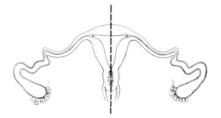

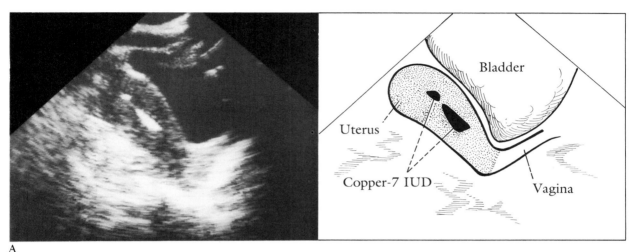

A

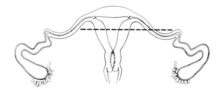

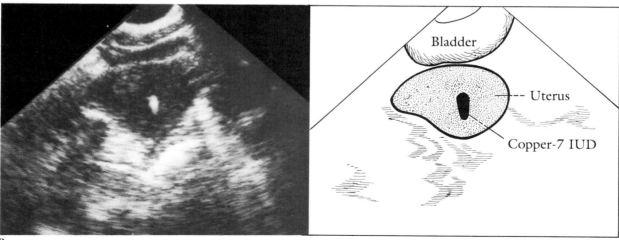

B

149

Fig. 4-39. The Dalkon Shield IUD could not be found during attempted removal. A. An ultrasound examination suggested that the IUD was in the right uterine wall.

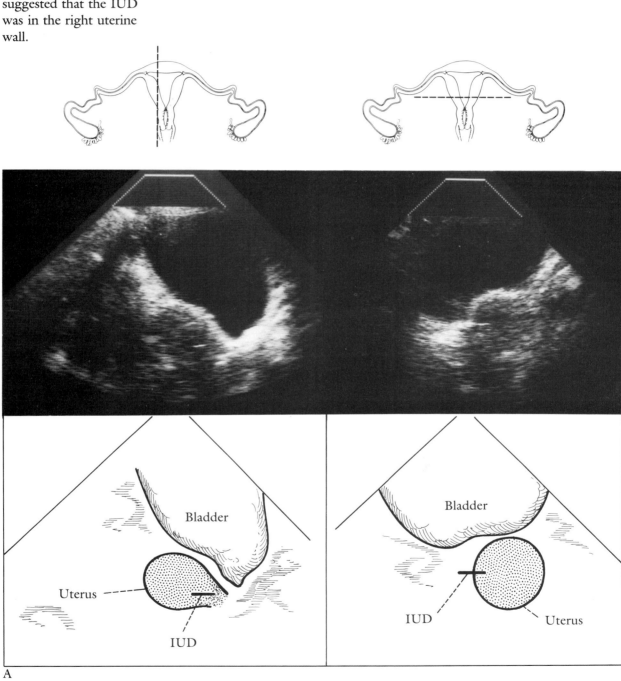

Bladder

Uterus

IUD

Bladder

IUD

Uterus

A

Fig. 4-39 (cont.)
B. Plain film of the pelvis showed the Dalkon Shield in the pelvis to the right of the intrauterine balloon catheter (*arrow*). C. On hysterosalpingogram the contrast outlined a normal uterine cavity and showed the IUD (*arrow*) well outside the cavity. At laparotomy the IUD was found buried within the right broad ligament.

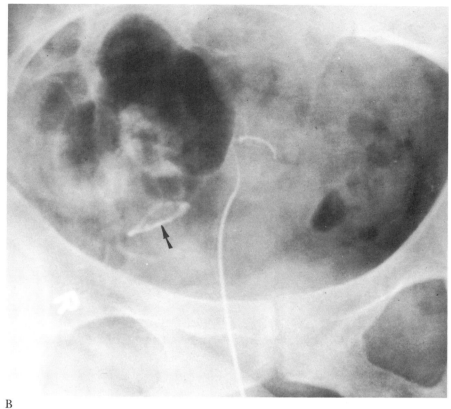

B

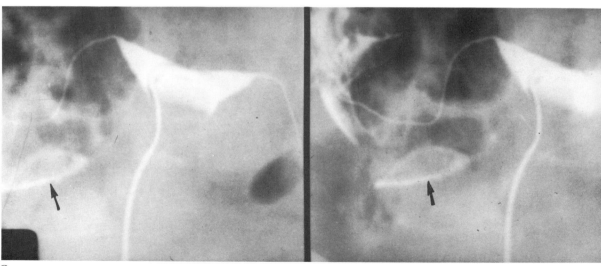

C

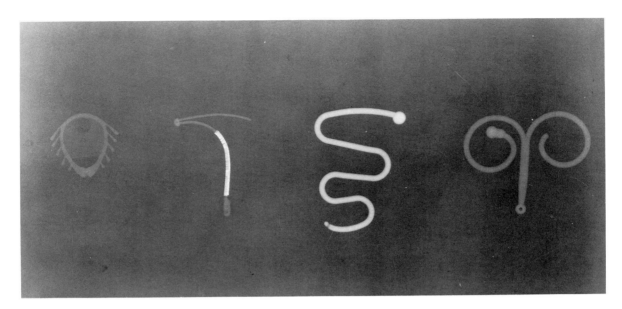

Fig. 4-40. Radiographic appearance of four intrauterine devices: (from left to right) Dalkon Shield, Copper-7, Lippes Loop, and Safe-T-Coil.

Once the IUD has perforated the uterus it may be difficult to find on ultrasound because the high-amplitude echoes are difficult to separate from pelvic fat and acoustic shadows created by air in the bowel (Fig. 4-39). In such cases a plain film of the abdomen is the next step. If the abdominal film shows absence of the IUD, its expulsion is confirmed. Dalkon Shields are faintly radiopaque and require careful scrutiny of the film and possibly coned-down views of the pelvis to exclude their presence (Fig. 4-40). If a pelvic IUD is seen on the abdominal film, hysterography is indicated. The plain film suggests perforation if the IUD is distorted, uncoiled, or rotated (Fig. 4-41), and the hysterogram verifies the position of the IUD outside the uterine cavity and serves as a guide to therapy [28]. Complete extension into the cul-de-sac is amenable to laparoscopic extraction. Partial perforation through the myometrial wall may indicate the need for laparotomy (Fig. 4-42).

An intrauterine pregnancy can occur next to a normally positioned IUD. On ultrasound it is easy to see the echogenic IUD adjacent to the gestational sac during the first trimester (Fig. 4-43). Later in pregnancy the IUD becomes harder to demonstrate. The IUD may be removed under sonographic monitoring, since its presence results in an increase of up to 50 percent in the rate of spontaneous abortion [31]. Ectopic pregnancy also occurs in IUD users and may be more common than in nonusers.

Fig. 4-41. A. Plain film of the pelvis showed a Lippes Loop IUD in an abnormal horizontal position. B. The hysterosalpingogram confirmed that the IUD was completely outside of the uterine cavity. Laparoscopic removal of the IUD from the cul-de-sac was easily accomplished.

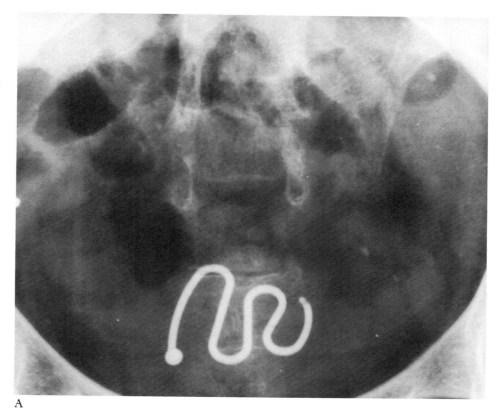

A

B

Fig. 4-42. A 40-year-old woman presented with pelvic pain and a metallic density seen on pelvic film. The hysterosalpingogram showed a piece of a Majzalin spring IUD (*arrow*) partially perforating the left uterine horn. The IUD had broken 5 years prior to the study during removal and bilateral tubal ligation.

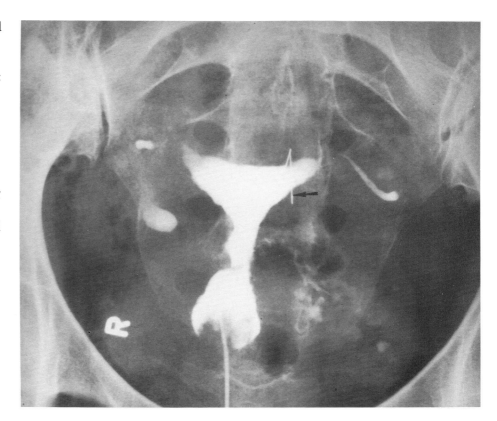

Fig. 4-43. A. Transverse view and

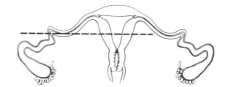

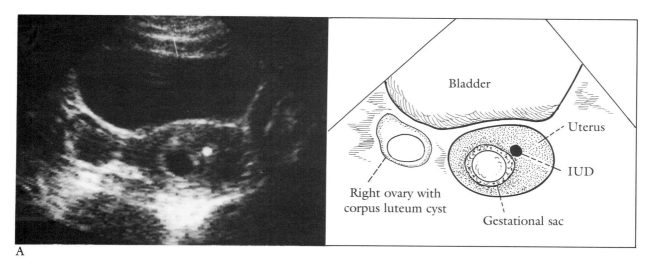

A

Fig. 4-43 (cont.)
B. two adjacent sagittal views of a pelvic ultrasound demonstrate an intrauterine device and an intrauterine pregnancy within the same uterine cavity. The patient had a Lippes Loop IUD inserted 19 months before the study. Her last menstrual period was 7 weeks prior to the study.

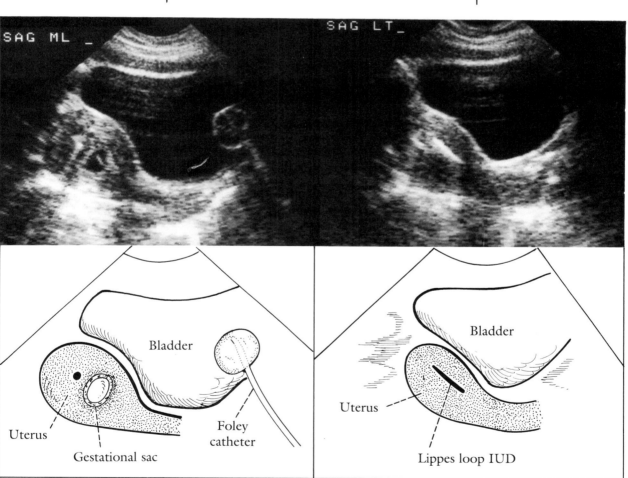

Bladder

Uterus

Gestational sac

Foley catheter

Bladder

Uterus

Lippes loop IUD

B

Fig. 4-44. Cesarean section scar. Hysterosalpingogram performed in a 34-year-old woman several years after cesarean section. Oblique view showed an anterior outpouching (*arrow*) at the level of the internal cervical os. Contrast filled a wide-mouthed diverticulum at the site of the cesarean section scar. A hysterosalpingogram prior to the cesarean delivery was normal.

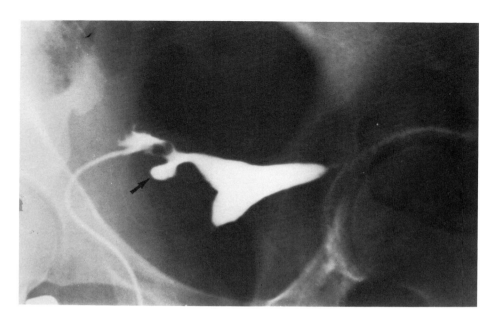

Cesarean Section Scar

Cesarean sections are usually performed by a low transverse incision of the uterine isthmus. Hysterosalpingogram may demonstrate the surgical site as a wedge-shaped or diverticular outpouching of the uterine cavity at the level of the internal os [43] (Fig. 4-44). These deformities may reflect a weakness at the surgical scar but their clinical significance is unknown.

References

1. Athey, P. A. Uterus: Abnormalities of Size, Shape, Contour and Texture. In P. A. Athey and F. P. Hadlock (eds.), *Ultrasound in Obstetrics and Gynecology* (2nd ed.). St. Louis: Mosby, 1985. Pp. 167–193.
2. Athey, P. A. Uterus: Abnormalities of the Endometrial Cavity. In P. A. Athey and F. P. Hadlock (eds.), *Ultrasound in Obstetrics and Gynecology* (2nd ed.). St. Louis: Mosby, 1985. Pp. 194–205.
3. Bates, G. W., and Wiser, W. L. Uterine Function and Abnormalities Causing Infertility. In J. Aiman (ed.), *Infertility, Diagnosis and Management*. New York: Springer, 1984. Pp. 143–160.
4. Bohlman, M. E., Ensor, R. E., and Sanders, R. C. Sonographic findings in adenomyosis of the uterus. *AJR* 148:765, 1987.
5. Breckenbridge, J. W., et al. Postmenopausal uterine fluid collection: indicator of carcinoma. *AJR* 139:529, 1982.
6. Buttram, V. C., and Reiter, R. C. *Surgical Treatment of the Infertile Female*. Baltimore: Williams & Wilkins, 1985. Pp. 201–228.
7. Cochrane, W. J. Ultrasonography and the intrauterine device. In W. B. Steel and W. J. Cochrane (eds.), *Gynecologic Ultrasound*. New York: Churchill Livingstone, 1984. Pp. 15–26.
8. Confino, E., et al. Sonographic imaging of intrauterine adhesions. *Obstet. Gynecol.* 66:596, 1985.

9. Daling, J. R., et al. Primary tubal infertility in relation to the use of an intrauterine device. *N. Engl. J. Med.* 312:937, 1985.

10. DeCherney, A., and Polan, M. L. Hysteroscopic management of intrauterine lesions and intractable uterine bleeding. *Obstet. Gynecol.* 61:392, 1983.

11. Dullea, G. Liability crisis complicates contraception. *N.Y. Times,* May 19, 1986. P. B8.

12. Fleischer, A. C., et al. Myometrial invasion by endometrial carcinoma: sonographic assessment. *Radiology* 162:307, 1987.

13. Gompel, C., and Silverberg, S. G. *Pathology in Gynecology and Obstetrics* (3rd ed.). Philadelphia: Lippincott, 1985. Pp. 149–277.

14. Gross, B. H., Silver, T. M., and Jaffe, M. H. Sonographic features of uterine leiomyomas: analysis of 41 proven cases. *J. Ultrasound Med.* 2:401, 1983.

15. Hall, D. A., and Yoder, I. C. Female Infertility. In J. F. Simeone (ed.), *Coordinated Diagnostic Imaging.* New York: Churchill Livingstone, 1984. Pp. 111–140.

16. Isaacs, I. Hysterographic double-outlined uterine cavity: a sign of unsuspected pregnancy. *AJR* 131:305, 1978.

17. Jones, H. W., and Seegar-Jones, G. Hyperplasia of the Endometrium and Endometrial Polyps. In *Novak's Textbook of Gynecology* (10th ed.). Baltimore: Williams & Wilkins, 1981. Pp. 377–390.

18. Jones, H. W., and Seegar-Jones, G. Endometrial Carcinoma. In *Novak's Textbook of Gynecology* (10th ed.). Baltimore: Williams & Wilkins, 1981. Pp. 391–426.

19. Kamal, I. *Atlas of Hysterographic Studies of the "IUD-holding Uterus."* Ottawa: International Development Research Centre, 1979. Pp. 23–67.

20. Malone, L. J., and Ingersoll, F. M. Myomectomy in Infertility. In S. J. Behrman and R. W. Kistner (eds.), *Progress in Infertility.* Boston: Little, Brown, 1975. Pp. 85–90.

21. March, C. M. Intrauterine and Cervical Pathology. In V. C. Buttram and R. C. Reiter (eds.), *Surgical Treatment of the Infertile Female.* Baltimore: Williams & Wilkins, 1985. Pp. 249–287.

22. Marshak, R. H., and Eliasoph, J. The roentgen findings in adenomyosis. *Radiology* 64:846, 1955.

23. Mischell, D. R. Current status of intrauterine devices. (Editorial.) *N. Engl. J. Med.* 312:984, 1985.

24. Norman, O. Hysterography in cancer of the uterus. *Semin. Roentgenol.* 4:244, 1969.

25. Olsen, A., and Christensen, P. Adenomyosis uteri diagnosticized by hysterosalpingography. *Fortschr. Rontgenstr.* 142:350, 1985. (In English).

26. Owolabi, T. O., and Strickler, R. C. Adenomyosis. A neglected diagnosis. *Obstet. Gynecol.* 50:424, 1977.

27. Pietila, K. Hysterography in the diagnosis of uterine myoma. Roentgen findings in 829 cases compared with the operative findings. *Acta Obstet. Gynecol. Scand.* [Suppl.] 5:1, 1969.

28. Rosenblatt, R., et al. Uterine perforation and embedding by intrauterine device: evaluation by US and hysterography. *Radiology* 157:765, 1985.

29. Schenker, J. G., and Margalioth, E. J. Intrauterine adhesions: an updated appraisal. *Fertil. Steril.* 37:593, 1982.

30. Sengupta, B. S., et al. Myomectomy in infertile Jamaican women. *Int. J. Gynaecol. Obstet.* 15:397, 1978.

31. Shalef, E., et al. Ultrasonically controlled retrieval of an intrauterine contraceptive device (IUCD) in early pregnancy. *J. Clin. Ultrasound* 15:525, 1987.

32. Siegler, A. M. *Hysterosalpingography* (2nd ed.). New York: Medcom, 1974. Pp. 82–95.

33. Slezak, P., and Tillinger, K. G. The incidence and clinical importance of hysterographic evidence of cavities in the uterine wall. *Radiology* 118:581, 1976.

34. Slezak, P., and Tillinger, K. G. The occurrence and significance of broad longitudinal folds in the uterine cavity at hysterography. *Radiology* 106:87, 1973.

35. Smith, J. P., et al. Ultrasonography of rapidly growing uterine leiomyomata associated with anovulatory cycles. *Radiology* 134:713, 1980.

36. Tak, W. K., et al. Myometrial invasion and hysterography in endometrial carcinoma. *Obstet. Gynecol.* 50:159, 1977.

37. Tristant, H., and Benmussa, M. *Atlas d'Hysterosalpingographie.* Paris: Masson, 1981. Pp. 119–129.

38. Tristant, H., and Benmussa, M. *Atlas d'Hysterosalpingographie.* Paris: Masson, 1981. Pp. 155–166.

39. Walsh, J. W., Taylor, K. J. N., and Rosenfield, A. T. Gray scale ultrasonography in the diagnosis of endometriosis and adenomyosis. *AJR* 132:87, 1979.

40. Walzer, A., Flynn, E., and Koenigsberg, M. Sonographic appearance of a prolapsing submucous leiomyoma. *J. Clin. Ultrasound* 11:101, 1983.

41. Weinstein, D., Arviad, Y., and Polyshuk, W. F. Hysterography before and after myomectomy. *AJR* 129:899, 1977.

42. Winer-Muran, H. T., Muram, D., and Gillieson, M. S. Uterine myomas in pregnancy. *J. Can. Assoc. Radiol.* 35:165, 1984.

43. Winfield, A. C., and Wentz, A. C. *Diagnostic Imaging of Infertility.* Baltimore: Williams & Wilkins, 1987. Pp. 127–157.

Chapter 5
Congenital Uterine Anomalies

Congenital anomalies of the uterus provide a fascinating subject for study. The incidence of congenital uterine abnormalities varies between 0.5 percent [14] and 1.0 percent [44] and depends on the method used for diagnosis. Uterine malformations are usually detected during manual inspection of the postpartum uterus, during hysterosalpingography, and during routine obstetric ultrasound examination. The hysterosalpingogram remains the most sensitive and accurate method of diagnosis. To a large extent uterine malformations stem from the total or partial failure of fusion of the paired müllerian ducts from which the uterus and fallopian tubes originate. Infertility is not often the presenting problem; instead these patients exhibit an increased number of obstetric complications. They experience more miscarriages; premature labor; fetal malpresentations, such as breech or transverse lies; than patients with a normal uterus and are therefore more likely to need a cesarean section.

Embryology

A brief review of the embryology is useful. The müllerian, or paramesonephric, ducts appear on the posterior abdominal wall of the 6-week-old embryo [40]. They develop as epithelial cords lateral to each mesonephric, or wolffian, duct. The müllerian ducts grow parallel to the mesonephric ducts, and canalization proceeds simultaneously with their downward growth [42]. On reaching the pelvic region, the müllerian ducts cross over the mesonephric ducts ventrally, approach each other in the midline, and fuse as they continue their caudal course [40]. The cranial unfused portions form the paired fallopian tubes; the caudal fused ducts form the uterus and cervix (Fig. 5-1). The caudal tip of the fused müllerian ducts, the müllerian tubercle, reaches the posterior wall of the urogenital sinus by the ninth week of development. In this region two outgrowths from the urogenital sinus, called the sinovaginal bulbs, proliferate rapidly and form the vaginal plate. By the fifth month the plate is elongated and canalized forming the vagina. As it canalizes, the vagina is lined by stratified squamous epithelium from the sinus [42]. The hymen, a transverse perforate membrane, forms where the vaginal plate meets the lower end of the urogenital sinus.

The uterus is derived from the fusion of the caudal part of the hollow müllerian ducts. At first the fusion between the ducts is incomplete, and a septum persists between the lumina [40]. Subsequent resorption of the median septum results in a single uterine cavity. Lack of fusion of the müllerian ducts, localized or throughout their entire length, explains the many different types of uterine duplications. Total or partial lack of resorption of the median septum accounts for the uterus septus and subseptus. The most common malformation is the uterus arcuatus, a minor lack of fusion of the uterine fundus [53]. The spectrum of malformations ranges from this mild deformity to the total failure of fusion seen in the uterus didelphys, which often coexists with a septate vagina. The unicornuate

Fig. 5-1. Embryology. The uterus and fallopian tubes develop from paired müllerian ducts.

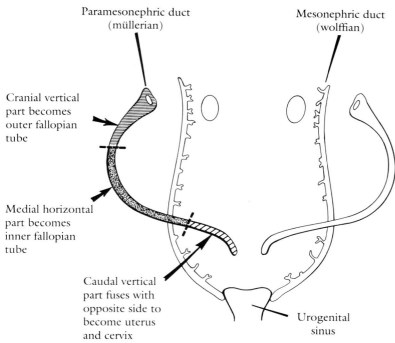

Paramesonephric duct (müllerian)

Mesonephric duct (wolffian)

Cranial vertical part becomes outer fallopian tube

Medial horizontal part becomes inner fallopian tube

Caudal vertical part fuses with opposite side to become uterus and cervix

Urogenital sinus

A

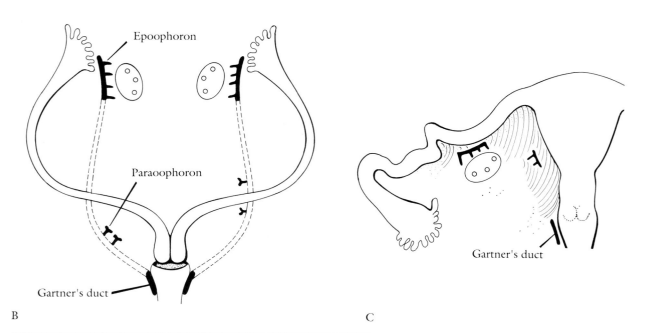

Epoophoron

Paraoophoron

Gartner's duct

B

Gartner's duct

C

uterus is a rare anomaly resulting from development of only one müllerian duct and varying degrees of atresia of the contralateral system. Aplasia of both müllerian systems leads to congenital absence of the uterus, usually accompanied by absence or shortening of the vagina.

Urinary tract abnormalities are often associated with genital malformations. The urinary and genital systems are derived from a common embryonic mesoderm, and it is easy to understand how an early teratogenic influence leads to defects in both systems. Over 50 percent of women with unilateral renal agenesis have reproductive tract anomalies and 20 percent of women with abnormal genital tracts have a urinary tract deformity, most commonly unilateral renal agenesis or renal ectopia [50]. Ultrasound provides the ideal diagnostic tool for simultaneous evaluation of the genital and the urinary tracts and most sonographers automatically examine both systems at the sign of a congenital abnormality in either [11].

Classification

In 1946 Jarcho [19] proposed a simple classification of fusion anomalies of the uterus that correlates well with the appearance of the uterine cavity as seen on hysterosalpingography. Figure 5-2 is an adaptation of Jarcho's classification expanded to include the communicating uterus [42] and uterine atresia [5]. The hysterosalpingogram can only be used in the diagnosis of uterine anomalies that communicate with the vagina. In the presence of vaginal obstruction or atresia ultrasound is the simplest way to examine the pelvic organs, but magnetic resonance imaging provides the best noninvasive demonstration of pelvic anatomy [43].

The classification of uterine anomalies (Fig. 5-2) is based entirely on the appearance of the uterus, but it is assumed that the user is familiar with the common associated vaginal anomalies. A sagittal septate vagina frequently occurs concurrently with a uterus didelphys and less often with a septate or bicornuate uterus. The vertical vaginal septum may be incomplete and cause one-sided genital obstruction with hematocolpos, hematometra, and hematosalpinx. Similarly uterine atresia is commonly associated with vaginal atresia or a transverse vaginal septum.

Duplicated and septated uterine cavities often communicate. The communication usually occurs in the region of the isthmus but may rarely be very low in the cervix. Toaff et al. [42] view isthmic communications as proof that embryologic resorption of the median septum begins at the isthmus and proceeds both cranially and caudally. If resorption of the septum is arrested in its first stage, there will be an opening between each uterine cavity at the level of the internal os.

Bilateral agenesis of the fallopian tubes has never been reported and unilateral tubal agenesis is seen only in association with a unicornuate uterus [5]. In utero exposure to DES causes uterine abnormalities that are not fusion defects and are categorized separately.

162   Congenital uterine anomalies

Fig. 5-2. Classification of congenital uterine malformations.

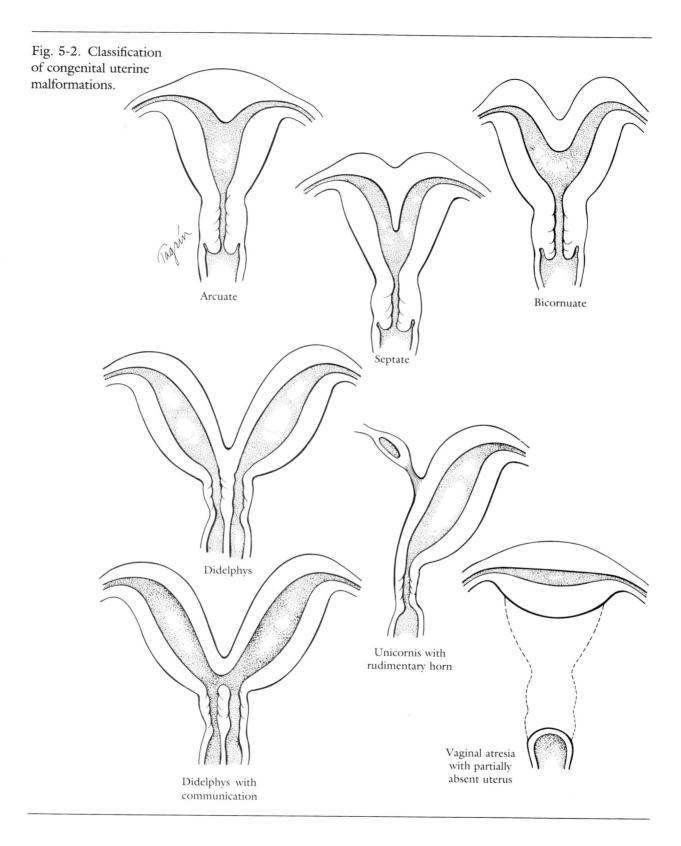

Arcuate

Septate

Bicornuate

Didelphys

Unicornis with rudimentary horn

Didelphys with communication

Vaginal atresia with partially absent uterus

Fig. 5-3. Arcuate uterus.
Normal hysterosalpin-
gogram shows a smooth
concavity of the uterine
fundus.

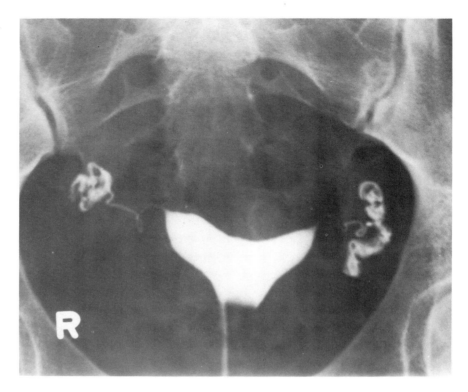

Arcuate Uterus

The diagnosis of an arcuate uterus is made incidentally during hysterography. Contrast in the uterine cavity demonstrates a concave indentation of the fundus instead of the normally convex or straight dome of the fundus (Fig. 5-3). The fundal concavity is smooth and shallow and easily differentiated from the V-shaped trough seen in a septate or a bicornuate uterus. A fundal myoma can indent the cavity of the fundus and simulate an arcuate configuration (Fig. 5-4). The arcuate uterus is such a minor deformity that it is considered a normal variant and is not associated with infertility or obstetric difficulties [44]. The fundal bulge of an arcuate uterine cavity decreases and alters the potentially available space for lodging an IUD [21]. The IUD may become compressed, distorted, or laterally rotated. This in turn increases pain, bleeding, and the possibility of expulsion of the IUD.

Sonographic diagnosis of a uterine malformation depends primarily on the detection of an abnormal external contour. The external contour of the arcuate uterus is normal; thus it is not recognizable by ultrasound [3].

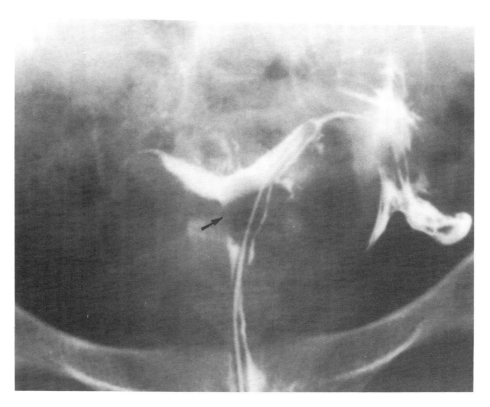

Fig. 5-4. Fundal myoma indents the superior aspect of the uterine cavity and mimics an arcuate fundus. The left tube is normal. The right tube has been surgically removed. The Foley balloon (*arrow*) is inflated within the uterine body.

Septate and Subseptate Uteri

Hysterosalpingography performed for the evaluation of recurrent abortion will demonstrate a 10 to 15 percent incidence of uterine duplication anomalies [27]. Septate and subseptate uteri are the leading causes of habitual abortion. The recurrent abortions may be caused by decreased cavitary volume or by inadequate blood supply of the uterine septum when the conceptus is implanted on the septum [5]. The more extensive the septum the greater the likelihood that it will be the site of implantation. The hysterogram demonstrates two separate and symmetric uterine horns in the septate uterus (Figs. 5-5 and 5-6) but cannot differentiate a septate from a bicornuate uterus. If the uterine horns are closely apposed with an acute angle between them a septate uterus is probable [38]. Laparoscopy demonstrates a shallow groove on the fundus of the septate uterus and a deep fundal cleft separating the two horns of the bicornuate uterus. The septum may be short and bisect only the fundus, or it may extend down to the isthmus and divide the uterus into two separate cavities with one cervix [6].

Sonographic demonstration of a uterine septum is only possible during pregnancy when the amniotic fluid allows visualization of the internal structure of the uterus [51]. During the second and third trimesters the septum appears as a linear echogenic structure extending from the fundus and separating the amniotic cavity into two parts. Characteristically fetal parts and activity are observed on both sides of the septum. In their series

Fig. 5-5. Septate uterus. The hysterosalpingogram shows two separate uterine horns in a 28-year-old woman who had two previous premature deliveries. There was a 60 degree angle between the uterine horns. A uterine septum was confirmed during cesarean delivery of third pregnancy.

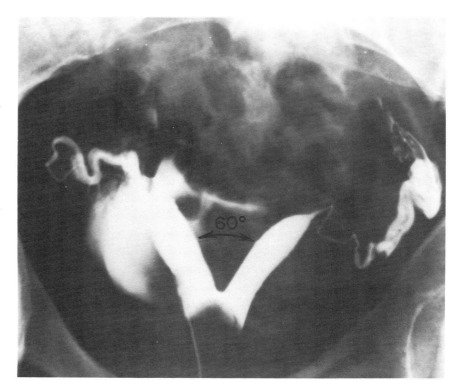

Fig. 5-6. Subseptate uterus. The hysterosalpingogram showed a shallow fundal indentation in a 26-year-old woman who had a 4-year-old child and three previous spontaneous abortions. A short uterine septum was noted at hysteroscopy.

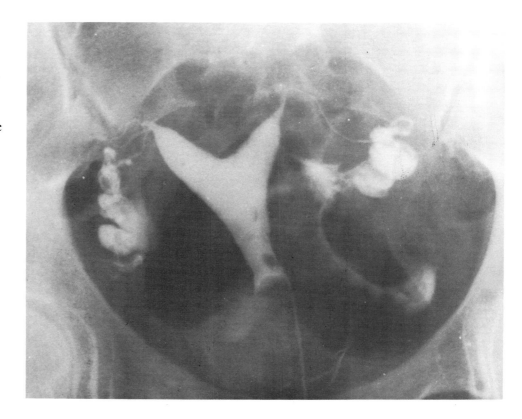

Worthen and Gonzalez [51] noted frequent placental implantation on the septum without evidence of placental insufficiency or fetal distress. They question whether poor vascularity of the septum results in fetal wastage and suggest future Doppler measurements of placental and septal blood flow in these cases. During obstetric sonography a uterine contraction in the fundus opposite the site of placental implantation or a cystic mass adjacent to the uterus may falsely suggest a uterine septum. However, the contraction is transient, and adjacent cystic masses lack fetal parts.

Patients with a septate uterus and habitual abortion may benefit from surgical correction by either the Jones wedge procedure [30] or the Tompkins metroplasty [27]. Both procedures report 70 to 80 percent successful pregnancy rates. The hysterogram after metroplasty shows marked reduction in the size of the uterine cavity and a narrow fundus with approximation of the tubal ostia [27]. More recently hysteroscopic resection of the uterine septum has been reported as a less traumatic surgical alternative that obviates the risk of peritoneal adhesions and increases the likelihood of subsequent vaginal delivery [6]. The hysterogram following successful hysteroscopic resection of the uterine septum demonstrates a completely normal uterine cavity.

Bicornuate Uterus

The bicornuate uterus is caused by a lack of fusion of the uterine body resulting in two separate uterine horns joined above one cervix (Fig. 5-7). On hysterography the diagnosis of a bicornuate uterus can be suspected when the contrast-filled horns are widely divergent and there is an obtuse angle between them [38] (Fig. 5-8). The bicornuate uterus may present such a striking hysterographic appearance that other uterine pathology such as a leiomyoma may be overlooked (Fig. 5-9).

On sonography the bicornuate uterus shows an expanded bilobed fundus with an echogenic endometrial cavity in each lobe [3] (Fig. 5-10). Ultrasound can also detect the two horns of a pregnant bicornuate uterus. Usually the pregnancy is located in one horn, and the other horn appears as an inferior mass with a prominent central hyperechoic region produced by the endometrial decidual reaction [25] (Fig. 5-11). The endometrial cavity echo allows recognition of the extra horn and prevents confusion with a uterine or ovarian mass. Rarely there is a pregnancy in each horn. The presence of two horns alerts the obstetrician to the many complications of such a pregnancy. The decidual membrane in the nonpregnant horn may be expelled, and vaginal bleeding may mimic an impending abortion or a placenta previa. The second horn may obstruct normal vaginal delivery and the majority of these patients will need a cesarean section. Several cases of repeated failed attempts at therapeutic abortion until an ultrasound examination demonstrated a bicornuate uterus and allowed selective evacuation of the pregnant horn have been reported [46].

Fig. 5-7. Bicornuate uterus. Laparoscopy in a 29-year-old woman showed a bicornuate uterus and no filling of the left tube with methylene blue. Physical examination revealed a single vagina and cervix. The hysterosalpingogram showed a short common cervical canal (*arrow*) and two separate uterine horns. Both fallopian tubes filled with contrast. During laparoscopy the Foley balloon used to infuse methylene blue had been inadvertently inflated in the right uterine horn, thus preventing infusion of left tube.

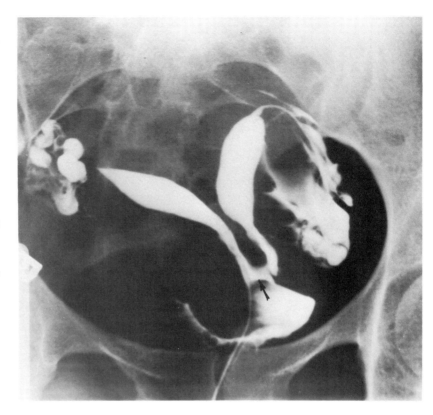

Fig. 5-8. Hysterosalpingogram in an infertile 25-year-old woman. A. The Foley balloon (*arrow*) was initially inflated within the left uterine horn and erroneously suggested a unicornuate uterus. (cont.)

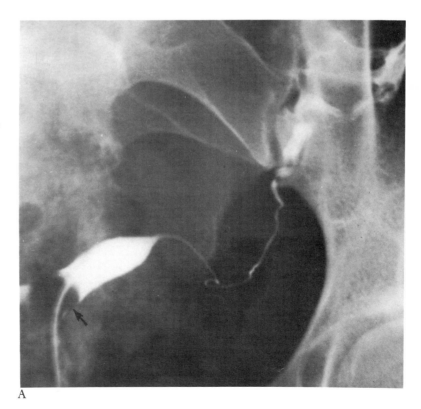

A

168   Congenital uterine anomalies

Fig. 5-8 (cont.). B. After the balloon was retracted into the cervical canal, a bicornuate uterus was seen with widely divergent horns. There was a 155 degree angle between the horns. Laparoscopy and hysteroscopy demonstrated the bicornuate uterus and bilateral pelvic kidneys.

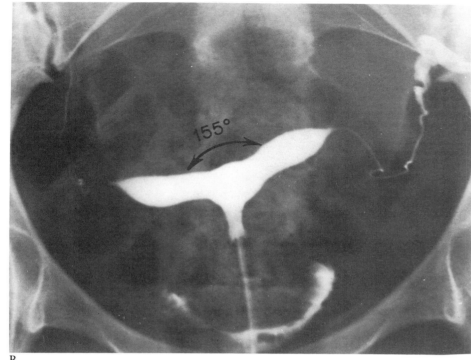

B

Fig. 5-9. A hysterosalpingogram was performed prior to myomectomy in a 26-year-old woman who, on the basis of a vaginal examination, was thought to have fibroids. A. Early and (B) late views showed widely divergent uterine horns and interstitial obstruction of the left fallopian tube. The configuration of the uterus was attributed entirely to a bicornuate uterus. At surgery both a bicornuate uterus and a 10-cm posterior fibroid were present. The fibroid was causing some extrinsic compression of the left horn. The left tube appeared normal.

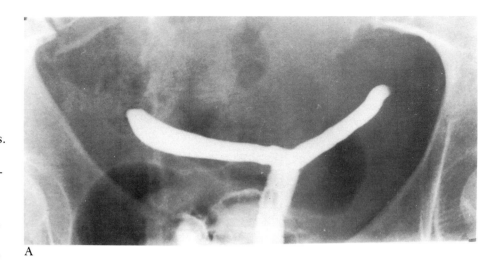

A

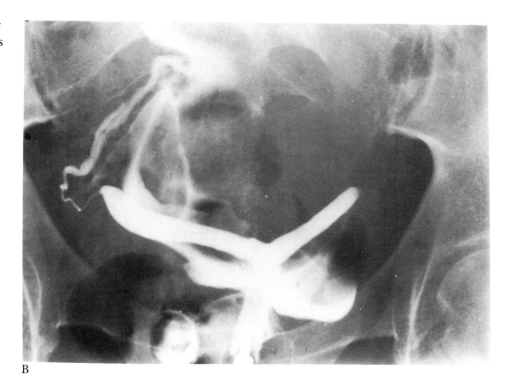

B

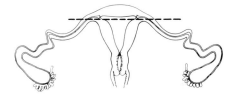

Fig. 5-10. Transverse sonogram of bicornuate uterus shows the two uterine horns. Each horn contains an endometrial cavity.

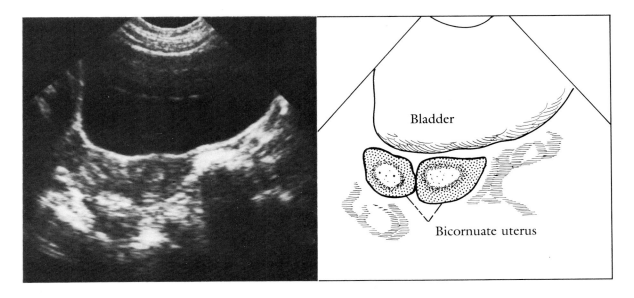

Bladder

Bicornuate uterus

Fig. 5-11. A. Transverse and (B and C) sagittal sonograms of a bicornuate uterus. There is an intrauterine pregnancy in the right horn, and an IUD and a prominent decidual reaction in the left horn. (Courtesy of Dr. Lucy Hann, Boston, Mass.)

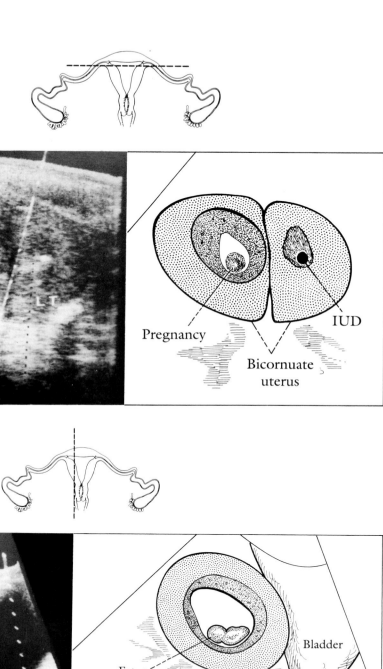

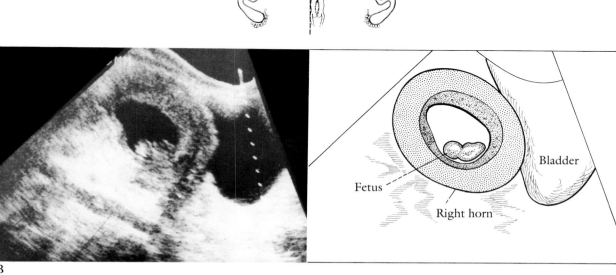

Fig. 5-17. Uterus didelphys. Sagittal sonograms through adjacent uterine bodies. A. The right uterine cavity exhibits a prominent decidual reaction. B. There was a 9-week pregnancy within the right uterine cavity. The patient miscarried several weeks later.

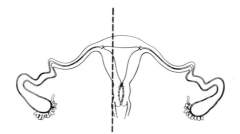

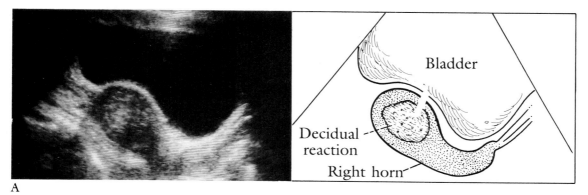

A

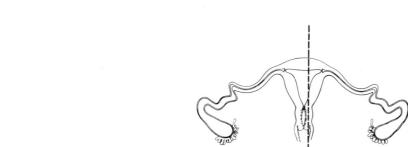

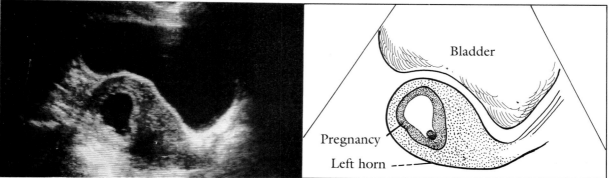

B

Unicornuate Uterus The unicornuate uterus is an uncommon abnormality created by development of only one müllerian duct. If the failure of the contralateral duct is incomplete, a rudimentary horn may be present with a fibrous connection to the unicornuate horn [49]. The rudimentary horn may have a small uterine cavity that seldom communicates with the unicornuate uterine cavity. The hysterogram of the unicornuate uterus demonstrates a single, tubular elongated cavity pointed toward the left or right side of the pelvis (Fig. 5-18). The appearance is identical to that of a single horn of a bicornuate uterus or one-half of a uterus didelphys. If the Foley catheter is introduced too far into the cervical canal of a bicornuate uterus, a unicornuate uterus may be falsely diagnosed. To prevent this occurrence careful study of the endocervical canal after partial deflation of the Foley balloon is recommended whenever a unicornuate system is found. Sometimes a normal uterus may mimic a unicornuate uterus when one of the tubes fails to fill with contrast. The midline position of the uterus, however, will suggest that it is not unicornuate, and oblique films will help delineate the normal fundus accurately.

The unicornuate uterus is difficult to demonstrate on ultrasound. A slender uterus displaced to one side may suggest its presence but is seldom diagnostic [11]. The contralateral rudimentary horn has never been demonstrated by ultrasound or hysterography.

Pregnancy in the rudimentary horn is a very rare event, but when it occurs it presents with the clinical symptoms of ectopic pregnancy and may lead to rupture of the horn. Pregnancy in the predominant horn requires careful sonographic monitoring because repeated abortions and severe intrauterine growth retardation occur frequently in patients with unicornuate uteri [1].

Fig. 5-18. Unicornuate uterus. A. The hysterosalpingogram showed a single left-sided uterine horn and fallopian tube. B. The Foley balloon was retracted to demonstrate the cervical canal and ensured that the balloon was not occluding a right-sided uterine cavity. Laparoscopy showed an atrophic right uterine horn with a tenuous fibrous connection to the normally developed left uterine horn.

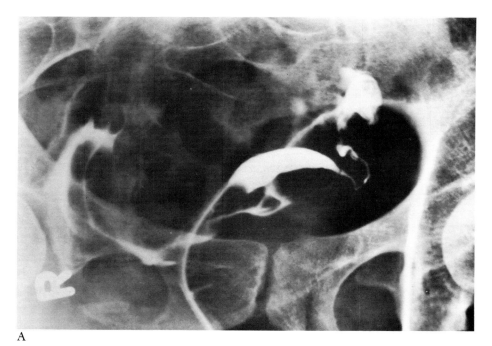

A

B

Unilateral Hematocolpos

Uterine failures of fusion and septation are frequently accompanied by a longitudinal vaginal septum. If the vaginal septum is incomplete, unilateral vaginal obstruction results. A review of the literature done in 1976 revealed a total of 41 cases of unilateral hematocolpos [52]. In that review all cases in which the urinary tract was investigated showed unilateral renal agenesis on the side of the obstructed hemivagina. Since then the number of reported cases has tripled and several patients have been found with normal kidneys [20,32]. Half a dozen cases have also been described with a dysplastic kidney and atretic ectopic ureter opening into the occluded vagina [12,13].

Unilateral hematocolpos presents in adolescents or young women with pelvic pain, menstrual irregularities, and a pelvic mass. A high index of suspicion and thorough preoperative investigation will prevent mutilating surgery [32]. Pelvic and renal ultrasound and hysterography are necessary for complete evaluation. Sonography reveals a midline cystic mass in the area of the vagina with variable extension into the pelvis. Ultrasound may also demonstrate separate uterine horns and dilatation of the obstructed side consistent with unilateral hematometrium and hematosalpinx [37].

The hysterogram is accomplished by introducing contrast into the patent cervix. The contrast delineates the extent of uterine duplication and may show a communication between the uterine cavities (Fig. 5-19) or between the uterus and the hematocolpos (Fig. 5-20). The communication allows partial decompression of the obstructed vagina but also serves as a source of contamination and infection of the old menstrual blood trapped in the hemivagina. In the absence of a communication it is possible to perform a transvaginal puncture of the obstructed side; aspirate some of its contents; and inject enough contrast to fill the vagina, uterus, and tube on that side [29].

Fig. 5-19. Hysterosalpingogram performed 7 months after surgical excision of an incomplete vertical vaginal septum and decompression of a right-sided hematocolpos, hematometrium, and hematosalpinx.

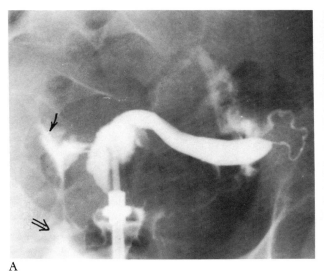

A

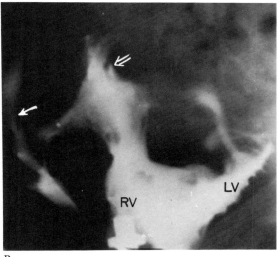

B

A. The left uterine horn and fallopian tube of a uterus didelphys appeared normal. There was a communication with the right horn (*solid arrow*) and duplicated vagina (*open arrow*) at the level of the cervical canal. B. The right uterine horn (*open arrow*) and tube (*closed arrow*) were dilated and deformed. Adequate filling of the right side was not achieved because the dilated cervical canal allowed free reflux into the right (*RV*) and left (*LV*) vaginal vaults. C. Drawing of right hematocolpos and communicating uterus didelphys prior to surgical excision of vaginal septum. (From I. C. Yoder and R. C. Pfister. Unilateral hematocolpos and ipsilateral renal agenesis: report of two cases and a review of the literature. *AJR* 127:303, 1976. Reprinted with permission.)

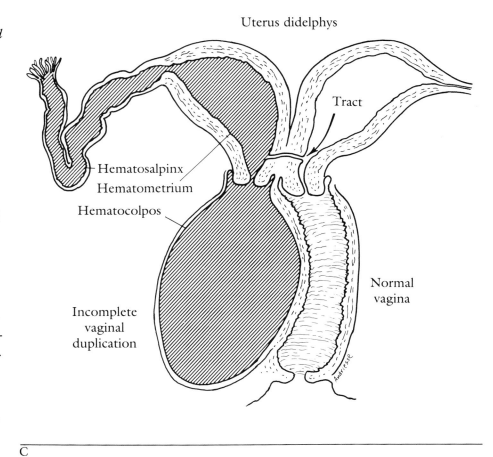

Uterus didelphys

Hematosalpinx

Hematometrium

Hematocolpos

Tract

Normal vagina

Incomplete vaginal duplication

C

181

Fig. 5-20. Hysterosal-
pingogram performed
prior to surgical decom-
pression of a right-sided
hematocolpos. A. Con-
trast instilled into a left
cervix filled a single
uterus (*U*) with evidence
of previous metroplasty
of a septate uterus. B. A
communication (*arrow*)
from the cervical canal
allowed contrast to
spill into the right
hematocolpos (*HC*). C
and D. Drainage views
in frontal and lateral
projections. Arrow
points to normal left
vagina. (*HC* = right-
sided hematocolpos; U
= uterus.) E. Drawing
of right hematocolpos
and communicating sep-
tate uterus. (From I. C.
Yoder and R. C. Pfister.
Unilateral hematocolpos
and ipsilateral renal
agenesis: report of two
cases and a review of the
literature. *AJR* 127:303,
1976. Reprinted with
permission.)

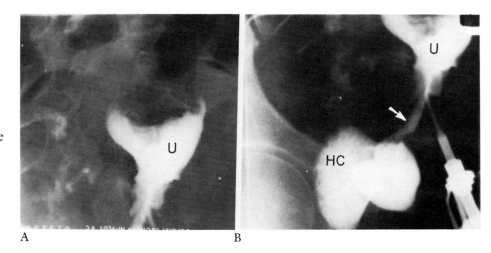

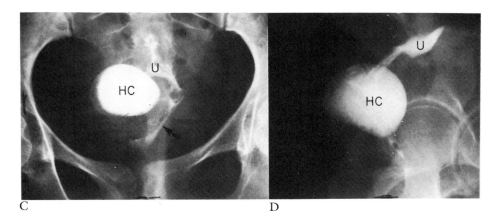

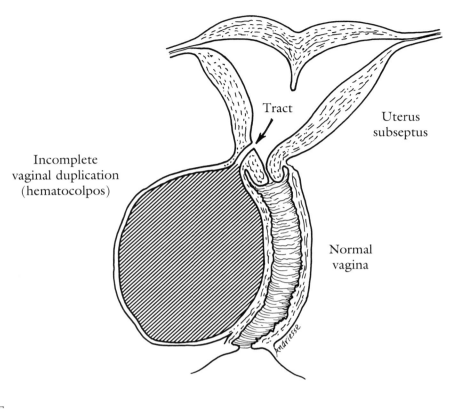

Fig. 5-20 (cont.)

Tract

Uterus
subseptus

Incomplete
vaginal duplication
(hematocolpos)

Normal
vagina

E

Excision of the vaginal septum usually leads to complete relief of symptoms and preserves reproductive capacity [35]. Unilateral hematocolpos must be differentiated from an imperforate hymen and a Gartner's duct cyst. Imperforate hymen results from lack of perforation of the transverse membrane that separates the vagina from the vestibule. Uterine and vaginal secretions cannot escape and cause hydrocolpos and bulging of the hymen. The problem is usually detected in infants and is not associated with other genital or urinary anomalies. Simple or multiple Gartner's cysts occur within the lateral uterine and vaginal walls and represent caudal remnants of the mesonephric duct that have failed to resorb normally in the female [48]. They may communicate with the lumen of the uterus, in which case they will opacify during hysterography and appear as thin tubular structures running parallel to the uterine cavity (Fig. 5-21) or the vagina (Fig. 5-22). A Gartner's duct cyst in the vaginal wall may have a sonographic pattern similar to that of a hematocolpos but is usually much smaller [26]. Ipsilateral renal agenesis may also occur with Gartner's duct cysts.

Fig. 5-21. Gartner's duct cyst. A. The hysterosalpingogram shows a linear cavity (*arrows*) parallel to the endocervical canal. B. The Gartner's duct cyst communicates with the uterine cavity and extends inferiorly (*arrows*) to end blindly alongside the vaginal vault. This was an incidental finding during a work-up for infertility.

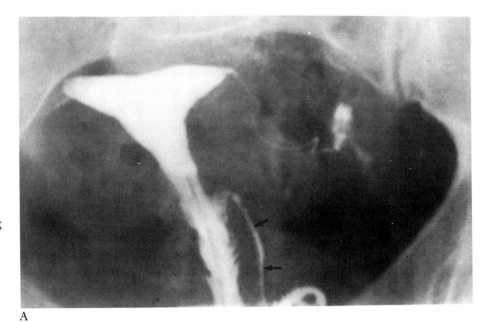

A

B

Fig. 5-22. Gartner's duct cyst. A. The hysterosalpingogram shows a tortuous linear cavity extending from the lower cervical canal and coursing horizontally along the vaginal vault (*arrows*). B. The Gartner's duct cyst continues inferiorly in a vertical course parallel to the vaginal wall (*arrows*). The vagina contains no contrast, but there is a large accumulation of contrast into the cul-de-sac (*CS*) from normally patent fallopian tubes.

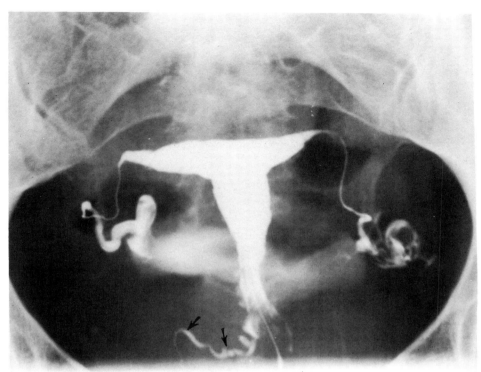

A

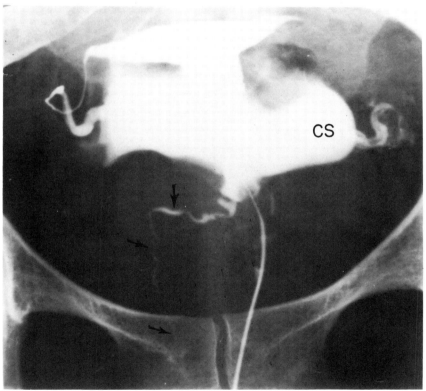

B

Vaginal Atresia

Congenital absence of the vagina and an abnormal or absent uterus (Mayer-Rokitansky-Kuster-Hauser syndrome) often coexist. While recognizing the contribution of all of the authors, Tarry et al. [41] suggest using a shortened version of this eponym. The Mayer-Rokitansky syndrome designates vaginal atresia with a spectrum of uterine anomalies ranging from a rudimentary uterine thickening to a normally developed uterus with an obstructed and dilated uterine cavity. The fallopian tubes and ovaries are usually normal. The patients are phenotypic females with a 46,XX karyotype and normal endocrine status.

Urinary tract abnormalities occur in 50 percent of patients with Mayer-Rokitansky syndrome and most frequently include unilateral renal agenesis or renal ectopia and less often horseshoe kidney or renal malrotation [36]. Skeletal abnormalities occur in 12 percent of patients; usually involve the spine; and include wedge vertebrae, fusions, and rudimentary or supernumerary vertebrae [36].

Patients with vaginal atresia present with primary amenorrhea and normal secondary sex characteristics. Hysterosalpingography is not possible. High-resolution sonography permits accurate preoperative scrutiny of the pelvic organs and simultaneous evaluation of the urinary tract. The ultrasound is performed with a tampon in the vaginal pouch and variable bladder filling [45]. The tampon identifies the vagina and facilitates measuring the distance between the vaginal apex and the lower uterus. Ultrasound also allows estimation of uterine volume. The uterus is usually atretic or there is localized cervical atresia with a normal fundus. Very rarely the uterus may be normal in shape but distended by trapped menstrual secretions.

When magnetic resonance imaging becomes widely available it will prove very useful in planning the surgical management of patients with vaginal atresia [43]. The sagittal magnetic resonance images unequivocally demonstrate the extent of vaginal and uterine development. Genital reconstruction depends on the extent of the abnormality with the best prognosis for fertility in those unusual patients who have a normal uterus above a partially atretic vagina. Patients with concomitant cervical and vaginal atresia have little likelihood of successful pregnancy. Early vaginal reconstruction and counseling may prevent adolescent emotional and behavioral problems.

DES Exposure in Utero

During the 25 years between 1945 and 1970, DES, a synthetic estrogen, was frequently prescribed for threatened abortion in the United States [8]. Smith and coworkers [39] at the Boston Lying-In Hospital provided the major stimulus for the drug's use despite a study by Dieckmann [9] in 1953 demonstrating that DES was ineffective in preventing miscarriages. In 1970 Herbst and Scully [17] reported six cases of clear-cell adenocarcinoma of the vagina in young women 15 to 22 years old. In 1971 Herbst et al. [18] linked the occurrence of these vaginal tumors to the maternal ingestion of DES during early pregnancy. That same year the Food and Drug Administration banned the use of DES in pregnancy. Initial fears of an epidemic of genital adenocarcinoma did not materialize. Although 1 to 2 million American women may have had in utero exposure to exogenous estrogen, the risk that these women will develop clear-cell adenocarcinoma is very low: It approximates 1 case per 1000 women from birth through 34 years of age [16]. The median age at diagnosis is 19 years, the range is 7 to 34 years. Through June of 1985 [28] a total of 519 cases of clear-cell adenocarcinoma of the vagina and cervix had been identified at the Chicago registry established to monitor the disease. In 72 percent of these cases the patient's mother received DES or other synthetic estrogen during pregnancy. The incidence of genital adenocarcinomas peaked in 1975 and has been declining since, but cases can be expected to occur until the year 2000 [28].

The malignant tumors attributed to DES are rare, and this suggests that the hormone is an incomplete carcinogen with other unknown factors contributing to the genesis of the tumors [16]. Far more commonly DES induces many unique benign changes in the female genital tract. It is postulated that DES crosses the placenta and exerts a target effect on the müllerian system of the fetus [34]. The drug inhibits the normal transformation of vaginal and cervical columnar müllerian epithelium into stratified squamous epithelium, and it produces vaginal and cervical adenosis as well as vaginal and cervical ridges in exposed women. These changes are most marked when large doses of DES have been given for a prolonged time very early in pregnancy. No müllerian duplication anomalies or urinary tract abnormalities have been associated with prenatal exposure to DES [24].

Vaginal adenosis is defined as the presence of glandular epithelium resembling endocervical or endometrial cells within the vaginal wall. Adenosis is the presence of normal tissue in an unusual location and does not require treatment because in most instances it disappears with time. Adenocarcinomas have been found adjacent to areas of adenosis, but the progression of adenosis to carcinoma has been difficult to document. Curiously, the gross structural changes of the cervix and vagina, such as ridges, hoods, and cock's combs, also decrease in size and may disappear during an extended period of observation [2].

Fig. 5-23. A young woman with documented exposure to DES in utero was undergoing an infertility investigation. The hysterosalpingogram demonstrated a T-shaped uterine cavity and a narrow lower uterine segment. There was a left hydrosalpinx (*H*) confirmed by laparoscopy.

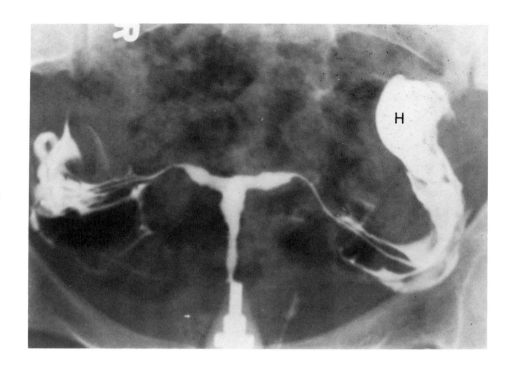

Hystero-salpingography

Any substance that produces visible changes in the cervix can by logical extension be expected to affect the remainder of the müllerian duct system [23]. Hysterosalpingographic examination of the uterus confirms this premise and reveals characteristic changes in the uterine cavity of DES-exposed women [23,31,33]. The most common abnormalities include: (1) a T-shaped uterine cavity accentuated by marked narrowing of the lower uterine segment (Fig. 5-23); (2) a widened boxlike lower cavity often accompanied by flaring triangular uterine horns (Fig. 5-24); (3) a general decrease in the size of the uterine cavity (Fig. 5-25); (4) annular constrictions of the uterine horns or body (Fig. 5-26); and (5) an irregular shaggy outline of the entire uterine cavity (Fig. 5-27). Uterine abnormalities are more common in patients with gross cervical and/or vaginal abnormalities and DES exposure during the first 12 weeks of gestation [23]. Women with abnormal uterine cavities are more likely to have a poor pregnancy outcome than DES-exposed women with a normal hysterogram. The T-shaped uterus, uterine constriction, and irregular margins are more frequently associated with infertility, ectopic pregnancy, and premature delivery, but a specific abnormality cannot be related to a specific pregnancy outcome [24]. These patients need careful monitoring during pregnancy with frequent ultrasound and cervical examinations. Cervical incompetence is sometimes present but cerclage is indicated only for the usual obstetric indications. Barnes [4] showed that among DES-exposed women who become pregnant 81 percent have at least one full-term live birth as compared with 95 percent of controls.

Fig. 5-24. Hysterosalpingogram in a 26-year-old DES daughter who had several first trimester miscarriages. The uterine cavity was characteristic of DES exposure in utero with irregular flaring of the cornua and a boxlike shape of the lower uterine segment. The right tube was normal, but the left tube showed an isthmic obstruction.

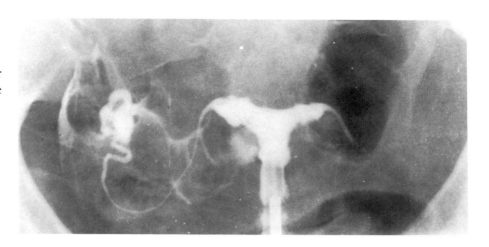

Fig. 5-25. Hysterosalpingogram in a 21-year-old DES daughter with 2 years of infertility. The uterine cavity was diffusely small and T-shaped.

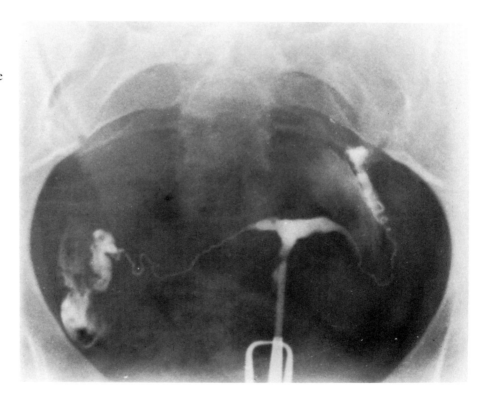

Fig. 5-26. Hysterosal-
pingogram in a young
woman with docu-
mented DES exposure
in utero. The uterine
cavity shows characteris-
tic annular constrictions
(*arrows*) of the uterine
horns.

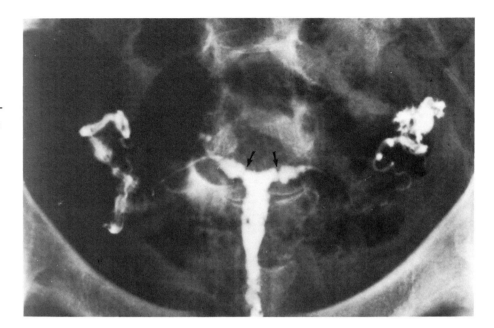

Fig. 5-27. Hysterosal-
pingogram in a DES
daughter shows a T-
shaped uterine cavity,
constriction of uterine
horns, and a shaggy out-
line of the entire uterine
cavity.

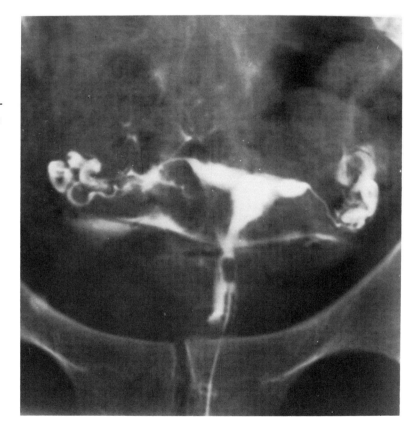

Fig. 5-28. A. Sagittal and (B) transverse views of a pelvic ultrasound show a nonspecific decrease in size of the uterus in a DES daughter.

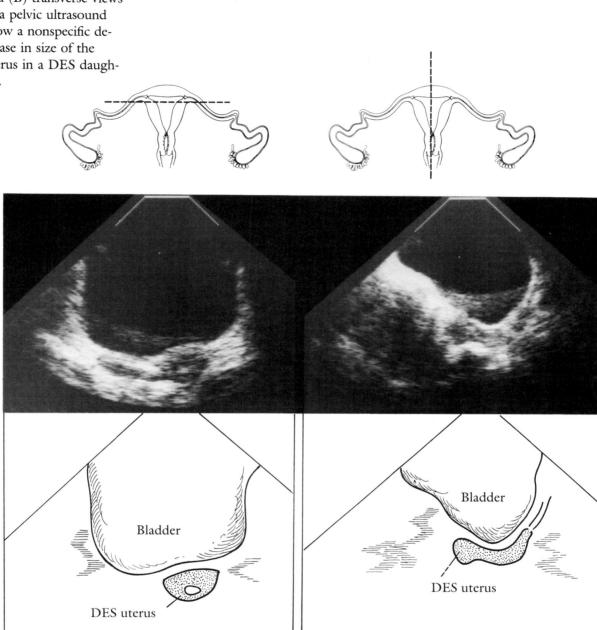

A   B

Fig. 5-29. Hysterosalpingograms performed on the hysterectomy specimens of four young women with adenocarcinoma of the vagina and documented DES exposure in utero. The uterine cavities in all specimens show characterisic changes: (A, B, and C) are T-shaped and (D) has a boxlike lower uterine segment. Pathologic examination of each uterus showed a generalized decrease in muscle mass to one-half of that usually found in normal menstruating women.

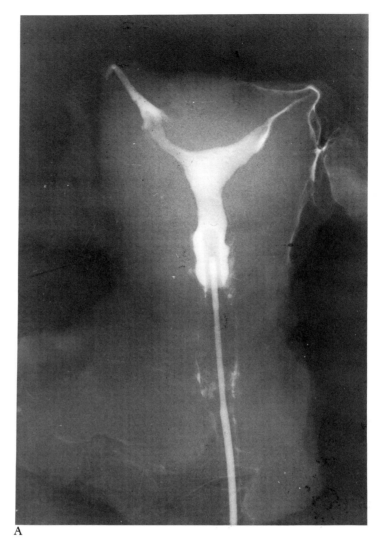

A

Haney et al. [15] used hysterosalpingography and a linear planimeter to show that the total area of the endometrial cavity is significantly smaller in DES-exposed patients compared with that of a control group undergoing routine infertility investigation. Uterine volume measured by ultrasound is also shown to be uniformly decreased to 50 cm³ in DES-exposed women (Fig. 5-28), compared with a 90 cm³ volume in normal subjects [47]. Pathologic examination of a small number of surgical specimens in DES-exposed women operated on for adenocarcinoma of the vagina shows a concurrent decrease in myometrial muscle to approximately one-half the muscle mass found in normal uteri (Fig. 5-29).

The differential diagnosis of a small T-shaped uterus includes an infantile uterus. In the infantile uterus the fundus and the cervix are roughly equal in

Fig. 5-29 (cont.)

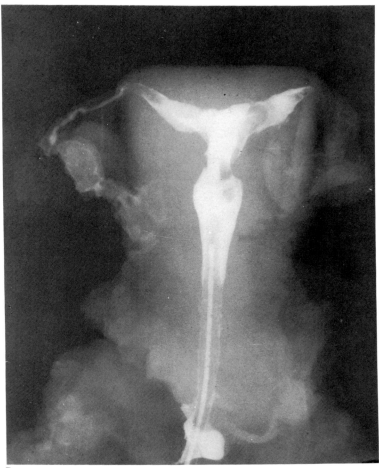

B

size, whereas in the adult uterus the fundus is 2 times larger than the cervix. The uterus acquires its adult proportions at puberty under the influence of endogenous estrogen. Adult women with severe estrogen deficiency may demonstrate small infantile-type uteri on the hysterosalpingogram (Fig. 5-30).

In 1981 DeCherney [7] offered the first and only description of abnormal fallopian tubes in 16 DES-exposed women undergoing studies for infertility. The tubes appeared normal on the hysterosalpingogram, but laparoscopic examination demonstrated foreshortened, thin-walled, and convoluted fallopian tubes with decreased fimbrial tissue and a pinpoint os in all cases. These so-called withered tubes may account for the increased incidence of infertility and ectopic pregnancy reported in some series of DES-exposed women.

Fig. 5-29 (cont.)

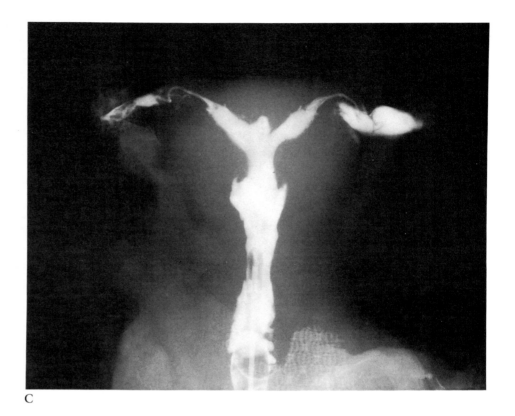

C

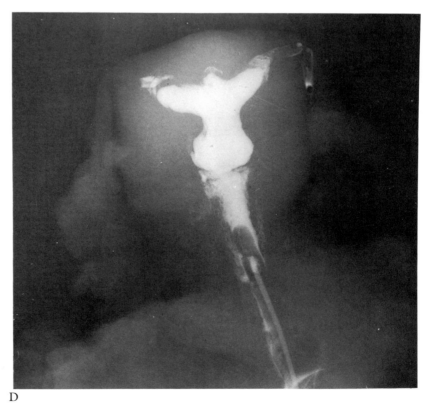

D

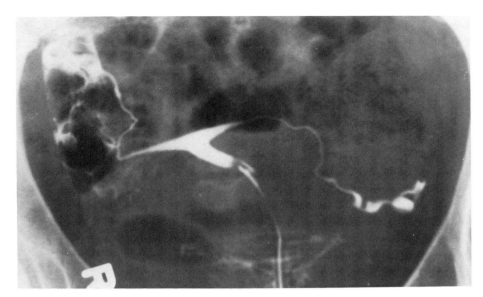

Fig. 5-30. The hysterosalpingogram in a 27-year-old woman with Kallmann's syndrome. There is a small T-shaped uterine cavity. The appearance is consistent with an infantile uterus. The uterus has not attained postpubertal proportions because of the absence of normal estrogen stimulus. (Kallmann's syndrome is a familial deficiency of leutinizing-releasing hormone and agenesis of the olfactory bulb. The patients present with primary amenorrhea and anosmia.)

Cervical Incompetence

Cervical incompetence is suspected when a midtrimester abortion occurs preceded by painless rupture of the membranes. The etiology of cervical incompetence is unknown and may be congenital or secondary to previous obstetric trauma. In the nonpregnant uterus the easy insertion of an 8-mm Hegar dilator and the demonstration of a widened internal cervical os on hysterosalpingography are considered diagnostic of cervical incompetence. The hysterogram shows a lack of normal internal os narrowing at the junction of the lower uterine segment and the cervical canal (Fig. 5-31). The abnormal internal cervical os measures more than 0.7 cm in diameter [22]. The x-ray magnification error can be corrected by comparing the width of the cervical os with that of the inner lumen of the Foley catheter [54].

Cervical incompetence is treated by suturing the cervix. Cerclage is performed during the first trimester of pregnancy. Obstetric ultrasound is routinely obtained prior to cerclage to assess the viability of the fetus. Ultrasound can also detect cervical os incompetence and provide objective criteria on which to base the need for cerclage. During first trimester sonography the incompetent cervix is shorter and the cervical os is wider than the normal competent cervix [10]. Prolapse of amniotic membranes into the cervical canal and vagina is easy to demonstrate (Fig. 5-32). Ultrasound also provides a convenient monitor of the effectiveness of cerclage (Fig. 5-33).

Fig. 5-31. Hysterosalpingogram in a 27-year-old woman who had several second trimester spontaneous abortions. The uterine cavity lacked a definite normal narrowing at the internal os. The narrowest part of the cervical canal (*arrows*) measured 11 mm. Subsequent pregnancy was managed with cervical cerclage and resulted in the delivery of a normal term infant.

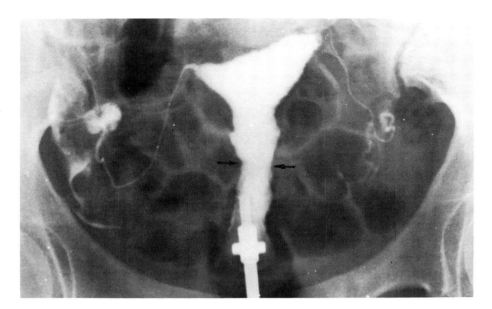

Fig. 5-32. A. Sagittal and (B) transverse sonograms in a pregnant woman show an incompetent cervix. The amniotic sac is bulging into an open cervical canal

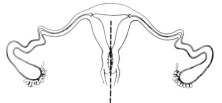

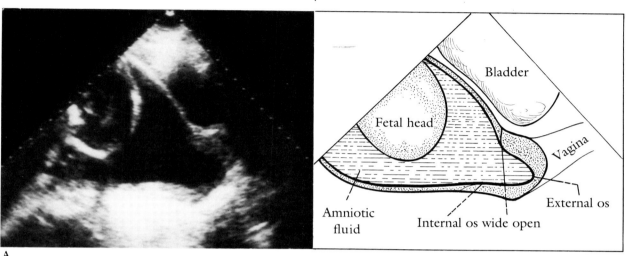

A

and the internal os is gaping. (Courtesy of Dr. Oksana Baltarowich and the Ultrasound Department of the Thomas Jefferson University Medical School.)

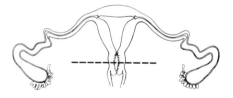

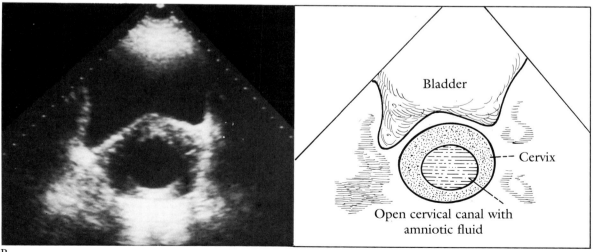

B

197

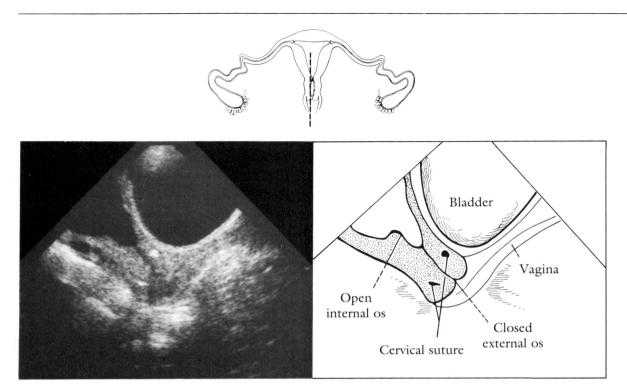

Fig. 5-33. Sagittal ultrasound in a pregnant woman with previous history of cervical incompetence. The amniotic fluid bulges into an open incompetent internal cervical os. The distal two-thirds of the cervix is closed and the cervical sutures are in place. (Courtesy of Dr. Oksana Baltarowich and the Ultrasound Department of the Thomas Jefferson University Medical School.)

References

1. Andrews, M. C., and Jones, H. W. Impaired reproductive performance of the unicornuate uterus: intrauterine growth retardation, infertility, and recurrent abortion in five cases. *Am. J. Obstet. Gynecol.* 144:173, 1982.

2. Antonioli, D. A., Burke, L., and Friedman, E. A. Natural history of diethylstilbestrol—associated genital tract lesions: cervical ectopy and cervicovaginal hood. *Am. J. Obstet. Gynecol.* 137:847, 1980.

3. Athey, P. A. Uterus: Abnormalities of Size, Shape, Contour and Texture. In P. A. Athey and F. P. Hadlock (eds.), *Ultrasound in Obstetrics and Gynecology* (2nd ed.). St. Louis: Mosby, 1985. Pp. 167–205.

4. Barnes, A. B., et al. Fertility and outcome of pregnancy in women exposed in utero to diethylstilbestrol. *N. Engl. J. Med.* 302:609, 1980.

5. Buttram, V. C., and Reiter, R. C. *Surgical Treatment of the Infertile Female.* Baltimore: Williams & Wilkins, 1985. Pp. 149–199.

6. Daly, D. C., et al. Hysteroscopic metroplasty: surgical technique and obstetric outcome. *Fertil. Steril.* 39:623, 1983.

7. DeCherney, A. H., Cholst, I., and Naftolin, F. Structure and function of the fallopian tubes following exposure to diethylstilbestrol (DES) during gestation. *Fertil. Steril.* 36:741, 1981.

8. DES Task Force Summary Report. Washington, D.C.: U.S. Department of Health Education and Welfare. Publication No. 79-1688, NIH, 1978.

9. Dieckmann, W. J., et al. Does the administration of diethylstilbestrol during pregnancy have therapeutic value? *Am. J. Obstet. Gynecol.* 66:1062, 1953.

10. Feingold, M., Brook, I., and Zakut, H. Detection of cervical incompetence by ultrasound. *Acta Obstet. Gynecol. Scand.* 63:407, 1984.

11. Fried, A. M., et al. Uterine anomalies associated with renal agenesis: role of gray-scale ultrasonography. *AJR* 131:973, 1978.

12. Gilsanz, V., and Cleveland, R. H. Duplication of the müllerian ducts and genitourinary malformation. Part I: The value of excretory urography. *Radiology* 144:793, 1982.

13. Gilsanz, V., and Cleveland, R. H. Duplication of the müllerian ducts and genitourinary malformation. Part II: Analysis of malformations. *Radiology* 144:797, 1982.

14. Green, L. K., and Harris, R. E. Uterine anomalies. Frequency of diagnosis and associated obstetric complications. *Obstet. Gynecol.* 47:427, 1976.

15. Haney, A. F., et al. Diethylstilbestrol-induced upper genital tract abnormalities. *Fertil. Steril.* 31:142, 1979.

16. Herbst, A. L., et al. Age-incidence and risk of diethylstilbestrol-related clear cell adenocarcinoma of the vagina and cervix. *Am. J. Obstet. Gynecol.* 128:43, 1977.

17. Herbst, A. L., and Scully, R. E. Adenocarcinoma of the vagina in adolescence. *Cancer* 25:745, 1970.

18. Herbst, A. L., Ulfelder, H., and Poskanzer, D. C. Adenocarcinoma of the vagina. Association of maternal stilbestrol therapy with tumor appearance in young women. *N. Engl. J. Med.* 284:878, 1971.

19. Jarcho, J. Malformations of the uterus. *Am. J. Surg.* 71:106, 1946.

20. Johnson, J., and Hillman, B. J. Uterine duplication, unilateral imperforate vagina, and normal kidneys. *AJR* 147:1197, 1986.

21. Kamal, I. *Atlas of Hysterographic Studies of the "IUD Holding Uterus"*. Ottawa: International Development Research Center, 1979. Pp. 23–67.
22. Kasby, C. B. Hysterosalpingography: an appraisal of current indications. *BJR* 53:279, 1980.
23. Kauffman, P. H., et al. Upper genital tract changes associated with exposure in utero to diethylstilbestrol. *Am. J. Obstet. Gynecol.* 128:51, 1977.
24. Kauffman, P. H., et al. Upper genital tract abnormalities and pregnancy outcome in diethylstilbestrol-exposed progeny. *Am. J. Obstet. Gynecol.* 148:973, 1984.
25. Kutcher, R., and Yee, J. M. Pelvic mass in late pregnancy, sonography of uterine duplication: report of two cases. *Am. J. Obstet. Gynecol.* 143:603, 1982.
26. McCarthy, S., and Taylor, K. J. W. Sonography of vaginal masses. *AJR* 140:1005, 1983.
27. McShane, P. M., Reilly, R. J., and Schiff, I. Pregnancy outcomes following Tompkins metroplasty. *Fertil. Steril.* 40:190, 1983.
28. Melnick, S., et al. Rates and risks of diethylstilbestrol-related clear-cell adenocarcinoma of the vagina and cervix. An update. *N. Engl. J. Med.* 316:514, 1987.
29. Miyazaki, Y., et al. Uterus didelphys with unilateral imperforate vagina and ipsilateral renal agenesis. *J. Urol.* 135:107, 1986.
30. Muasher, S. J., et al. Wedge metroplasty for the septate uterus: an update. *Fertil. Steril.* 42:515, 1984.
31. Nunley, W. C., Pope, T. L., and Bateman, B. G. Upper reproductive tract radiographic findings in DES-exposure female offspring. *AJR* 142:337, 1984.
32. Pinsonneault, O., and Goldstein, D. P. Obstructing malformations of the uterus and vagina. *Fertil. Steril.* 44:241, 1985.
33. Rennell, C. L. T-shaped uterus in diethylstilbestrol (DES) exposure. *AJR* 132:979, 1979.
34. Robboy, S. J. A hypothetical mechanism of diethylstilbestrol (DES)-induced anomalies in exposed progeny. *Hum. Pathol.* 14:831, 1983.
35. Rock, J. A., and Jones, H. W. The double uterus associated with an obstructed hemivagina and ipsilateral renal agenesis. *Am. J. Obstet. Gynecol.* 138:339, 1980.
36. Rosenberg, H. K., et al. Mayer-Rokitansky-Kuster-Hauser Syndrome: US aid to diagnosis. *Radiology* 161:815, 1986.
37. Rosenberg, H. K., et al. Duplication of the uterus and vagina, unilateral hydrometrocolpos, and ipsilateral renal agenesis: sonographic aid to diagnosis. *J. Ultrasound Med.* 1:289, 1982.
38. Siegler, A. M. *Hysterosalpingography* (2nd ed.). New York: Medcom, 1974. Pp. 61–81.
39. Smith, G. V., and Smith, O. W. Prophylactic hormone therapy: relation to complications of pregnancy. *Obstet. Gynecol.* 4:129, 1954.
40. Snell, R. S. *Clinical Embryology for Medical Students* (3rd ed.). Boston: Little, Brown, 1983. Pp. 215–243.
41. Tarry, W. F., Duchett, J. W., and Stephens, F. D. The Mayer-Rokitansky

syndrome: pathogenesis, classification and management. *J. Urol.* 136:648, 1986.

42. Toaff, M. E., Lev-Toaff, A. S., and Toaff, R. Comunicating uteri: review and classification with introduction of two previously unreported types. *Fertil. Steril.* 41:661, 1984.

43. Togashi, K., et al. Vaginal agenesis classification by MR imaging. *Radiology* 162:675, 1987.

44. Tulandi, T., Arronet, G. H., and McInnes, P. A. Arcuate and bicornuate uterine anomalies and infertility. *Fertil. Steril.* 34:362, 1980.

45. Valdes, C., Malini, S., and Malinak, L. R. Sonography in the surgical management of vaginal and cervical atresia. *Fertil. Steril.* 40:263, 1983.

46. Valdes, C., Malini, S., and Malinak, L. R. Ultrasound evaluation of female genital track anomalies: a review of 64 cases. *Am. J. Obstet. Gynecol.* 149:285, 1984.

47. Viscomi, G. N., Gonzalez, R., and Taylor, K. J. W. Ultrasound detection of uterine abnormalities after diethylstilbestrol (DES) exposure. *Radiology* 136:733, 1980.

48. Wepter, J. F., and Box, R. M. Mesonephric duct remnants (Gartner's Duct). *AJR* 131:499, 1978.

49. Whitehouse, G. H. Congenital Abnormalities of the Female Genital Tract. In *Gynaecologic Radiology*. London: Blackwell, 1981. Pp. 56–72.

50. Winfield, A. C., and Wentz, A. C. *Diagnostic Imaging of Infertility*. Baltimore: Williams & Wilkins, 1987. Pp. 45–62.

51. Worthen, N. J., and Gonzalez, F. Septate uterus: sonographic diagnosis and obstetric complications. *Obstet. Gynecol.* 64:34S, 1984.

52. Yoder, I. C., and Pfister, R. C. Unilateral hematocolpos and ipsilateral renal agenesis: report of two cases and a review of the literature. *AJR* 127:303, 1976.

53. Zarretti, E., Ferrari, L. R., and Rossi, G. Classification and radiologic appearance of the upper cervical canal in women with a history of premature delivery. *J. Reprod. Med.* 30:677, 1985.

54. Zlatnik, F. J., et al. Radiologic appearance of the upper cervical canal in women with a history of premature delivery. *J. Reprod. Med.* 30:677, 1985.

Index